An Alzheimer's Guide

Activities and Issues for People Who Care

by Pat Nekola

Revised 2007 Applewood Ink
a division of: Catering by Design

Second Edition

ISBN: 0-9660610-9-8

Library of Congress Cataloging Number: 2001088548

Published by:
Applewood Ink
A division of: Catering by Design
P.O. Box 181
Waukesha, WI 53187

Dedication

I would like to dedicate this book to
my mother, Mary V. Evans,
and my aunt Genevieve (Gene).
Both women suffered and died with the Alzheimer's Disease.

May they happily dance
with the angels in heaven
as they rest in peace.

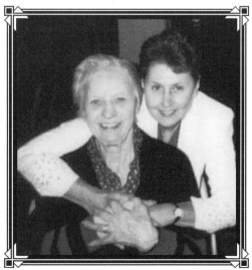

Pat and her mother after lunch at the hospital during
her mother's testing.

Contents

Part One:
Activities and Issues for People Who Care

Part Two:
Activities for Alzheimer's Patients

Introduction

I taught school for 15 years and ran a catering service for 18 years. I became very interested in learning about Alzheimer's when my own mother was diagnosed. I placed my mother into an independent living arrangement for one month and then a group home. It did not take me very long to understand she could no longer function in an independent living facility. She needed more care. I visited her daily and spent many hours with her. I made her needs known to the people in charge at the group home.

I read the information suggested by the social workers about the disease. I called the Alzheimer's Association to find out more about how to use their library. I began attending the group sessions they provided. I talked to doctors, nurses, and social workers to try to get help and good care for my mother. Eventually, I joined an advocacy group and attended monthly meetings for about a year. I also participated in the Memory Walk, sponsored by the Alzheimer's Association, in honor of my mother.

I attended counseling meetings to help me cope with my family's difficulty in deciding what was in Mom's best interest. I began to document my mother's actions and words to help me understand my situation better.

I started out by focusing all of my efforts and energy on my mother's care. But as time went on I realized that there was a much bigger picture for me.

Through my observations of my mother and other residents with dementia, I became very interested in finding activities to help the residents feel good for the moment. Mom was in the second stage of Alzheimer's at that time. She could still crochet a little, peel vegetables, dress herself, and do simple tasks with cues. Her judgement was very poor and her cognitive ability was deficient. She needed help for her daily care, hygiene, and management of her financial affairs.

When my husband and I first brought Mom to Wisconsin and placed her at the independent living facility, we did not realize that the disease had progressed as far as it had. It wasn't that I was in denial about Mom's disease, though that is a problem for many adult children. Like most people, I just was not knowledgeable about Alzheimer's. It is a progressive mental disease that strips the person of a sound mind, and families do not know how to read the situation. Some families have a feeling of helplessness and hopelessness. Often family members react out of fear or guilt when there is a diagnosis of Alzheimer's. Guilt, in particular, is apparent among adult children.

A social worker suggested that we take Mom to the Senior Health Center at the local hospital to have her tested. Test scores were very low for Mom's mental status. She also was tested at a later date and the doctor stated that she could not remember the day, month, time, nor the year. It became clear to me that Mom had Alzheimer's after several doctor appointments. I had Mom tested several times because other family members were denying Mom's condition.

At that point I was staying with her day and night at the independent living facility. I got home companions to come in to help care for Mom to give me short breaks for respite care. Another meeting was held at the independent living setting with a team of social workers and a nurse. They encouraged me to move Mom to a group home. I found a list of names of group homes to visit. After looking at fifteen homes, we placed Mom in one we knew would be appropriate for her.

She had her own private room. She needed that privacy, yet she had other seniors around her. She had the funds to take care of her health needs plus excellent health insurance benefits. It was an adjustment for Mom and our entire family. I watched Mom sit by the fireplace in a large wing-back chair. She'd never had a fireplace in her home. She loved the warmth and quietness at night. She talked to me about having three good meals and peaceful surroundings. She looked forward to our short rides in the country and trips to the ice cream parlor. It was a time of my life in which I learned a great deal about my mother even though she was living in her own little world. Through all the trials and tribulations I have some fond memories that I hold in my heart which spur me on in my daily living to help other Alzheimer's patients and their family members.

My Aunt Gene also had Alzheimer's. My uncle passed away after living in a nursing facility with Aunt Gene in northern Indiana. My cousin also brought her mother to Wisconsin. My aunt was much farther along in the disease than my mother was at the time. Aunt Gene was very docile while many times Mom was combative. I also learned much about the disease from my visits to Aunt Gene in the nursing home. While visiting the facilities I realized that activities were so vital to help sustain the Alzheimer's patients' well-being. I decided to go back to school and become certified as an activity director. I accomplished my goal in 1998, and continued to take my ideas and implement them in various care facilities in the Milwaukee area, and other parts of the country. As I saw how my ideas worked on the Alzheimer's patients, I began to document them. That documentation eventually evolved into this book.

In the second part of the book I have included activities involving stories, music, art, colors, parties, cooking, history, gardening, exercise, and nature that are very appropriate for Alzheimer's residents. Music is the rhythm to the inner spirit. Through music many residents respond in a positive manner. It is one of the greatest tools used to interact with the elderly population in general. Also, most folks like to eat and have parties because family celebrations were a part of their lives in the past.

When I was a teacher I told stories to get my point across to my high school students; I decided to apply that technique to my Alzheimer's program. I used cooking and baking to make the activity areas smell good and also to perk up the olfactory sense to help the participants stay alert. Like my mother, many residents have lost track of the month and time. Bright colors also help to stimulate residents. My aunt loved bright colors.

For almost 25 years I did not play my accordion. One day I decided to get the old accordion out and practice. I sounded very rusty. I said, "I can do this if I try." Just then I remembered my dad telling me, "If you can dream it, you can do it." His words spurred me on. I continued to practice until the songs came back to me. I took my accordion to the facility where Aunt Gene was staying and played many old-time songs. The residents enjoyed this greatly. I had many decorations from my catering company stored in my basement. I thought, I can set up a simulated party and talk about it with the residents. Then I decided to play music to the theme of the party. In addition I dressed up like Betsy Ross to do a mini-play with the residents. After the play I played patriotic songs on the accordion honoring the spirit of 1776 and Independence Day. Many residents played rhythmic instruments, waved flags, and hummed along with the music. After trying out my idea I saw the success of this activity and continued to add other activities to my program. Colorful flags and rainbows also attract the attention of the residents. My purpose in doing activities is for the residents to have fun, relax, and have a sense of belonging in the group. Through my activities with the residents I have developed a sense of trust, friendship, and love.

God gives love to people that truly love the elderly. To touch an elderly person's life is God's precious gift. From my commitment to serve the elderly I have been blessed and rewarded over and over. The elderly have given me many beautiful moments and the benefits of warmth and love. I use the accordion as a tool as part of my hour-long programs as I travel to the facilities and reach out to the Alzheimer's patients, interweaving topics of interest to the residents.

Activities in this book are designed for the month and season of the year. I have been able to implement the activities in various care facilities. I have enjoyed the responses—facial expressions, eye contact, hugs, and holding hands. I have laughed and cried with them. People ask, "How can you work with Alzheimer's patients?" I respond, "It is God's work. Where can you give and receive so much love in return for the interaction with God's beautiful people?"

Disclosure

I do not proclaim to be an expert in Alzheimer's. I am not trained in the medical field, nor am I a lawyer.

I became interested in Alzheimer's because my mother and aunt both suffered from the disease. I read every article I could find on the subject. I attended a support group for families of Alzheimer's patients, and then trained to become a co-facilitator for a support group in my community. I took a class in estate planning at the Waukesha County Technical College in Waukesha, Wisconsin. I also took caregiving classes in 1996, completed 90 hours of study in the activity consultants and trainers program in 1997, and 90 hours of study in management activity in 1998. These courses trained me to run activities in a care facility. At that point I began to gather information for this book.

I have experience in working with the elderly in several care facilities, and was an activity director for a year. Since 1995, I have worked with Alzheimer's patients, directing activities and living for the moment with these great people.

I have traveled around the country doing book signings for my *Picnics: Catering on the Move* cookbook, talking with families about the loss of a loved one to AD while raising funds for various local Alzheimer's Association chapters. I have listened to their stories; I've laughed and cried and exchanged hugs with many of them. We share a bond of both pain and joy.

I've combined my studies with my practical hands-on experience and the stories I've heard into this book, hoping to reach out to others dealing with Alzheimer's. I hope to help families, caregivers, and laypersons to cope with the disease. For me, the hardest part was losing my mother and aunt twice—first to the disease and then to death.

I hope you will read this book and apply the information to your situation, to help enrich the life of a loved one with Alzheimer's and to help you cope with your loss.

Part One

Activities
and
Issues for
People
Who Care

Chapter 1:

Understanding the Disease

The Four Stages of the Disease

Alzheimer's disease is an irreversible, progressive, and incurable disease that causes changes in the brain cells, a form of dementia that causes loss of memory.

Dr. Alois Alzheimer, a German physician, first talked about changes in the brain we now call Alzheimer's disease. Though the disease doesn't affect any two people in exactly the same way, there are four distinct stages of Alzheimer's that patients pass through.

- The First Stage is marked by short-term memory loss. While a person can still remember things from years before, he/she can't remember what happened five minutes ago. Judgment becomes impaired. Patients may believe they ate lunch or took their medication when they didn't. People with this disease are good fakers, especially with their adult children. A long-distance phone call to Mother or Dad is not very revealing. They may act like everything is all right because they fear losing their independence or becoming a burden on other family members. A person in the beginning stages of Alzheimer's may blame the memory problem on stress, or on other people. As the disease progresses, personality changes occur: withdrawal, anger, combativeness. It is painful for family members to watch these changes in a loved one.

- In Stage Two, patients have more difficulty in processing and remembering new information or following a story. They may be more sensitive to noise and less tolerant of young people. Simple hygiene needs are neglected. Long-term memory remains intact, however. They can still converse about familiar topics such as the weather, and they can still respond to instructions with cues.

∎ In Stage Three, the disease's symptoms become much more pronounced and the disease becomes fully evident to family and friends. Patients may wander off without a coat in the dead of winter, or eat 25 cookies and not remember doing so, or put the iron in the freezer. They need help with the simplest tasks of personal hygiene. They forget to pick up their feet when walking, and begin shuffling when moving about. They may not always recognize family members, or may confuse them, thinking their son is their husband, for example.

∎ In Stage Four, patients no longer even recognize their own faces in the mirror, much less those of family members. They are unable to express pain or feelings. They forget how to chew; all foods must be pureed and spoon-fed. They can no longer control bladder and bowel functions. They respond only to tactile stimuli, and, becoming bedridden, may revert to the fetal position. The brain slowly continues to shut down. The length of time a person lives with Alzheimer's can be as long as twenty years, but the median is eight years. In general, the younger the person is at the onset of the disease, the more quickly it progresses.

Many Potential Causes, But No Cure

There are many ideas and theories about the cause of the disease, but so far there is no cure. Researchers can't point to one factor. The apoE4 gene on chromosome 19—one form of the apoE gene which produces the protein apolipoproteinE4—has been linked to late-onset Alzheimer's. It occurs in about 40 percent of all late-onset patients. Adults who inherit two apoE4 genes (one from each parent) are at least eight times more likely to develop the disease than people who have two or more of the more common E3 version. There also have been studies that show that women who take estrogen replacement after menopause have lower rates of Alzheimer's disease than those who do not.

With new testing techniques, it is possible to learn a person's genetic makeup. Is this wise? It is understandable that a person would want to know as much as possible about his/her future. But there are real risks to that knowledge. If a person is tested and the gene is present, insurance companies may deny coverage, and there is the emotional toll of worry and fear over something that may never occur.

(My advice? Don't get tested. Just be prepared for old age by having your estate in order, your health care power of attorney and financial power of attorney assigned, your will and living will completed, your guardian selected, and your life, in general, in order. By age 85, fifty percent of people have Alzheimer's or some other form of dementia. Take life one day at a time, and live your life to the fullest.)

Important Signs To Be Aware Of

Family members often wait far too long to help their loved one with Alzheimer's for they themselves are not prepared to see the signs. Many adult children attribute Mom or Dad's forgetfulness to old age. It is true that there are various causes of memory loss: sometimes people seem disoriented when they are depressed, inebriated, or malnourished. Others have difficulty with the regulation of the thyroid. It is always best to schedule a checkup with the family doctor when chronic memory loss is noticed. If the problem worsens, it may be necessary to see a neurologist, neuropsychologist, or a geriatric psychiatrist. They will want to know the history of the patient's decline, to do a full medical exam, and to administer mental status tests to provide a baseline. A follow-up visit is usually recommended within two months. Don't let it go past six months. There are many changes that can take place in a couple months' time.

Multi infarc dementia (MID) is caused by a series of "mini-strokes." My mother had many of these mini-strokes, which contributed to her dementia. High blood pressure, high cholesterol, heart disease, and diabetes can all cause strokes, though each can be controlled by medication. Early diagnosis is important; at the beginning stages, medications can slow the progression of the disease. Talk to the doctor about the benefits and possible side effects of these drugs.

Apraxia and the Alzheimer's Patient

Apraxia is the loss of memory of how to perform complex muscular movements. It can be baffling to the caregiver who doesn't understand how the disease affects the brain. When the patient, for example, asks for a drink of water, the caregiver may reply, "Why, Mom, the water is in front of you." The patient may ask again for a drink. The caregiver must stop what he/she is doing, go to the patient, pick up the glass of water, place it in the patient's hands, and help him or her drink the water. This may need to be done many times, because the patient will not remember.

If a caregiver notices Dad sitting in the dark, he/she may explain how to open the blinds. The next day, he/she may scold the patient for not opening the blinds. "I told you yesterday how to open the blinds!" But you cannot expect him to remember from one day to the next, or even minute-to-minute, how to do a task. That part of the memory is gone.

Another resident with Alzheimer's that I worked with could do small tasks with help. If I put a peg into her hand, she could put it into a hole. With my cues, she could do the task.

Aphasia and the Alzheimer's Patient

Aphasia is the partial or complete loss of the ability to use or understand words. A patient with aphasia may still be able to participate in conversations and activities as long as he/she is asked yes/no questions. A person with aphasia does not necessarily have Alzheimer's. While working in a nursing facility, I got to know a woman who had aphasia. She was very sharp. Though she could not speak, she could nod and shake her head yes and no. She loved the music I played for the patients. She was always glad to participate in the activities I led for the residents.

Ways to Cope

Usually, at the onset of the disease, people do not realize that they have a memory loss problem. When they start to realize that there is something wrong, they may become very frustrated, anxious, or withdrawn and depend on others around them to "cover" for them. One of the best things you can do at this point is to help with practical needs: keeping track of time, people, places, and appointments. Here are some helpful tips for the person who is dealing with this stage of the disease.

If You Have a Family Member in the Early Stages of Alzheimer's, Give Him or Her This List and Help Them to Implement It.

❏ Have a book of important notes with you wherever you go. It should list phone numbers of family members, your own phone number and address, a list of appointments, a map of your own home, and your thoughts or personal reminders to help you function.

❏ Write important phone numbers, including emergency numbers, in large print and place them by the telephone. Put your address near the telephone as well.

❏ Use an answering machine to help you keep track of your messages.

❏ Get a large-print calendar and mark off each day to keep track of the date.

❏ Get a clock with large numbers that tells you both the date and time, and put it in a prominent place.

❏ Put pictures up on the cupboard door to list the contents.

❏ Ask a friend or relative to stop in and check to see that you eat and take your medications. As the disease progresses, it will become necessary to have someone else verify that you are taking your medications properly. Otherwise, you may mix up the medicines, take them twice, or skip taking them altogether.

❏ Organize your medications in pill boxes to help remind you when to take pills.

❏ Keep photos of loved ones you see regularly nearby so that you see them frequently. Write the names on each photo so you can put names and faces together.

❏ If you have trouble remembering the way to the grocery or other once-familiar places, take another person along with you.

❏ Let people know you have memory loss.

❏ If you are prone to wandering, register with the Alzheimer's Association's Safe Return program.

❏ Attend an Alzheimer's support group.

❏ Keep a daily routine.

❏ Converse in a place free of noise and large crowds.

In the beginning stages, patients will have good days and bad days. They may not be able to do things that once gave them pleasure or let them maintain their independence like bake homemade bread, balance a checkbook, or take a walk. As they deal with their memory impairment, don't let them be hurried by anyone. If something is too difficult, make sure they swallow their pride and ask for help.

There are people who feel embarrassed by memory loss and withdraw from friends and activities. It is important that they explain to people that they have memory loss. I once defended a neighbor with impaired memory when her husband made fun of her. She frequently repeated things and had difficulty remembering. I told him that he needed to help her by learning about the disease and giving her his support. He did come around, but it wasn't easy for him, either. He too felt the pain of losing her and had his own anger to deal with.

If your loved one is dealing with beginning-stage Alzheimer's disease, make sure they take some precautions with their overall health. Help them to:

- ❏ Stay physically fit. Exercise (with a doctor's approval).
- ❏ Stay in a safe environment.
- ❏ Take a break and relax if they are tired.
- ❏ Eat well-balanced meals.
- ❏ Don't drink alcoholic beverages—they only worsen memory.
- ❏ Take their medicine.
- ❏ Keep their stress levels to a minimum.

Safety First

People who are dealing with the advanced stages need to be especially careful of safety issues. Their judgment becomes poor. They may do things that put themselves, or others, in danger. They should not live alone. They should not be allowed to drive when it is no longer safe for them to do so. Their small appliances should have automatic shut-off devices and they should install an adequate number of smoke detectors. They must be cautioned never to let anyone in the house that they don't recognize.

There are many early-stage Alzheimer's patients who can live on their own successfully. This can happen when the doctor and family members stay involved and step in when necessary. Being educated about the disease helps a patient, and his or her family, to be better prepared for the way the disease progresses, and gives the family a better idea of how they can help.

My Own Experience

My mom always seemed very strong and independent. I learned much from watching her in her business. I would never have imagined her as an Alzheimer's patient.

Like many people, we were slow to pick up on the signs. A neighbor of hers reported that when she was riding with Mom to the local grocery store, Mom couldn't remember the way. The neighbors had also seen her walking up and down the street in her nightgown at 2 p.m. When I went to visit Mom, I found rotten food in the refrigerator, and her house was infested with mice and roaches. She roamed around the house at night and kept me awake. I realized that she wasn't herself any longer, that she was in trouble.

At first my mother could express her fears to me about losing her memory. She held her own for a year. Then she took a big dip again, and she steadily declined from there. She had lucid moments almost to the end of her life.

One of the things my mom worried about at first was what her future held for her. She didn't want to leave her home after 55 years. It was heartbreaking to have to remove her from there, and I waited too long to do it.

For Mom, like many others, the disease was overwhelming and frustrating. "I am going crazy!" she would yell. "Yes, I am going crazy!" She would scream and cry and stomp her feet. "I am crazy and I am worthless." I would swallow hard and say, "No, Mom, you are not crazy. I love you, and I'm here for you every step of the way." When she said that she should just die and then it would be all over, I would tell her that God wanted her here on earth with our family.

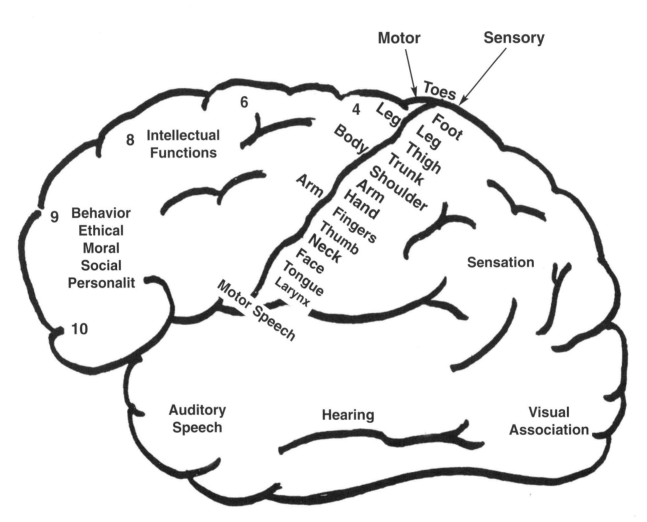

This is an example of the brain and how it guides our body to function daily.

The emotions were intense. She sometimes felt a great deal of anger and would act out. She sometimes felt lonely or very sad, which she expressed to me. I tried hard to lift her spirits. For her, a ride in the country was particularly soothing. I kept my sense of humor with Mom and could sometimes get her to laugh along with me. There are medications available to ease the feelings of sadness; if their sorrow is overwhelming, talk to a doctor about whether those would be helpful.

Mom also expressed her frustration at the changes in her life and said she felt guilty when she needed to ask for help. She had always kept everything "in her head," and never needed to write down reminders. She had always been the one who had taken care of everyone else all her life, the type of person who never asked for anything.

Professional help and family counseling helped me to understand Mom's disease. I worked hard to follow the advice of the counselor, who told me to enjoy those precious moments with Mom when she was lucid.

As Mom got worse, she lost a lot of weight. On one of my visits she did not recognize me. I carried on a simple conversation, talking about old times. She sometimes would whisper a few garbled words in return. The counselor told me that it was impossible to know what she could understand or what she was thinking.

Three weeks before she passed on, I held her frail body in my arms, stroking her face and brushing her hair. I prayed the rosary and sang some of her favorite songs as she laid very still. I bent down and kissed her and said, "I love you, Mom." She responded clearly, "I love you too, honey." I praised God for that precious moment. It is a gift I will hold in my heart forever.

For More Information

■ If you want to learn more about the brain, you can obtain copies of *On the Brain*, and *Brain Work: The Neuroscience Newsletter*. Write to the Charles A. Dana Foundation, 1001 G Street NW, Suite 1025, Washington, DC 20001-4545, for your free copies.

■ ADEAR, the Alzheimer's Disease Education and Referral Center, is a national resource center, and publishes *Connections*, a quarterly newsletter for professionals. Write ADEAR, P.O. Box 8250, Silver Spring, MD 20907-8250, or call (800) 438-4380.

■ The National Institute on Aging (NIA) leads the federal effort on aging research. Write NIA, Building 31, Room 5C27, Bethesda, MD 20892, or call (301) 496-1752.

■ The Alzheimer's Association (www.alz.org) is a great source of information. It is also responsible for the Safe Return Program launched in 1993. Every chapter of the Alzheimer's Association has help lines and a library to reach out to the patient and the family. The number for their headquarters is (800) 272-3900.

■ There is a wealth of information available on the Internet. One site I recommend is http://webmd.lycos.com. It features an Alzheimer's Disease Information Center.

Chapter 2:

Estate Planning and Other Legal Issues: A Priority

The importance of estate planning cannot be overstated. For a person with an Alzheimer's diagnosis, it is more important than ever, because the quality of care he/she will receive during the later stages of the disease may depend on the legal and financial documents that exist once the person can no longer make decisions for themselves.

My husband and I took a six-week course at a local technical college that helped us understand how to prepare for our retirement. If you want your wishes to be known and carried out, getting things on paper and legally in order is a must—while you are "of sound mind." Select an attorney who specializes in estate planning, probate, and elder law. A person who has complicated financial matters needs to make sure that every detail is covered. Without the proper documentation, you may be at the mercy of a guardian that the court chooses, who may or may not carry out your wishes.

No matter how small or large your estate, you should make this a priority. It is also important to have funeral arrangements in order, and your wishes regarding burial, cremation, and funeral services in writing.

I know of a situation where a man who had not seen his aunt in 30 years showed up to visit her after she was placed in a nursing home, suffering from advanced-stage Alzheimer's. Of course she didn't recognize her nephew. After her death, her estate went through probate court. On the day her will was read, her nephew went to court, stood up and asked if he was in the will. He was, after all, "the favorite nephew." Upon learning that he received nothing, he became disruptive. Having your legal documents in order protects you from a bunch of "favorite nephews" claiming a part of your estate after your death.

A Checklist if you Have a Loved One
With an Alzheimer's Diagnosis

❏ Attend Alzheimer's Association support meetings and educational programs that deal with legal issues.

❏ Consult an attorney who specializes in elder law, estate planning, and probate. Legal issues are complex and require the attention of a knowledgeable professional.

❏ Check your loved one's life insurance policies for a disability premium waiver.

❏ Check into organizations to find out if the person is entitled to any assistance.

❏ If the person, or the person's spouse, is a veteran, call the Veteran's Administration at (800) 827-1000 to check on eligibility for a disability pension.

❏ Help your loved one to make a list of assets and the form of ownership.

❏ Get him/her to update their will and estate matters.

❏ If appropriate, help him/her to apply for Social Security disability payments.

❏ Monitor the amount of cash the person carries. Take control of all credit cards and the checkbook.

❏ If you are the caregiver, consider what the future holds as the disease progresses. Caring for a person with Alzheimer's is very expensive, and being responsible for the disbursement of a person's funds is a difficult task. As the disease progresses, it may be necessary to consider a nursing facility. If you can afford private-pay facilities, there are many that are specially designed for Alzheimer's patients. Continue to educate yourself about community resources and make choices early to help ease the transition.

The above list is taken from a newsletter from Indianapolis Alzheimer Chapter. I found this list to be most helpful while assisting in my mother's care.

Protecting Your Funds When You are in Mourning

When your loved one—especially a spouse or parent—dies, it is a very hard time. You should not make any hasty financial decisions from six months to a year after the person's death. Get professional help and advice from an accountant and/or a lawyer to be on the safe side. When someone you love dies, you may go through emotions such as anger, loneliness, confusion, and fear. This makes you very vulnerable and you may make some bad financial judgments. Even an accountant who is very good at numbers isn't him- or herself when they lose a spouse or a parent. Safeguard all of your assets until you can better concentrate on the finances when you are more emotionally stable. My personal financial advisor told me to keep in mind the following points:

- Do not spend your money on frivolous items.
- Do not invest your money in risky stocks or junk bonds.
- Do not sell or remodel your home. (It is wise to stay put for one year after your loved one's death.)
- Don't make any purchase that exceeds five percent of your net worth.
- Keep your same job unless you absolutely cannot.
- Don't take financial advice from a well-meaning friend or relative. Get professional help.
- Don't pay off your mortgage.
- Don't borrow money if at all possible.
- Don't lend or give away your money to friends and relatives.
- Invest for safety, simplicity, and flexibility. When investing make sure that you utilize only federally insured banks, credit unions, or savings and loans institutions. Be sure you do not invest in a get-rich scheme with your inheritance and be very cautious about investments. Establish spending in moderation. Live within your means. Set a budget and know where your money is going for the year and years ahead.

For More Information

For further information on legal issues, contact your attorney. If you do not have an attorney, contact your state or local Bar Association for a referral to an attorney who is experienced in elder law, estate planning, and probate.

Chapter 3:

How the Disease Affects the Family

The Emotional Roller Coaster Ride

When a loved one is diagnosed with Alzheimer's, family members have different reactions.

What did I do wrong?

How could this happen to someone I love so much?

I am so angry. How could this happen to me?

I don't want to believe it. Can we get a second opinion?

What should I and my family do now that we know it is Alzheimer's?

Family members' responses can be negative: denying, rejecting, disagreeing, resenting, blaming, fearing, overreacting, withdrawing. Or they can be positive: accepting, loving, collaborating, listening, advocating, honoring, understanding, preparing, caring, learning, helping, organizing, sharing, educating, considering, consoling.

Anger

People who get angry with their loved ones with Alzheimer's need to understand their anger and reconsider their thinking. When someone stays angry it can be harmful not only to the Alzheimer's patient but to the caregiver and to the other family members as well.

Fortunately, I wasn't angry toward my mother once the doctor confirmed a diagnosis of Alzheimer's. But I have witnessed anger in other caregivers and have heard many unfortunate stories while traveling the country.

One woman told me she had too many unpleasant responsibilities and she was angry because she couldn't cope with her situation.

Many people are angry because they feel unappreciated for their efforts. For instance, a woman named Marilee told me she had the unpleasant chore of taking her mother out of her home. Her mother was verbally abusive toward her daughter because of this, even though Marilee was doing all the things the doctor had suggested, for the safety and best interests of her mother. Every time Marilee would visit, her mom would scream and shake her fist at her, accusing her of stealing all her worldly possessions, of not loving her, and of being a bad daughter. Marilee felt terrible about the situation until she got counseling and gained the affirmation that she was really doing the best that a daughter could do for her mom. Marilee got some training on how to cope with a mentally ill parent. That training helped her to accept her mom's anger without getting angry herself.

Another woman I met said that her family did not give her much support or show any appreciation for all her hard work while caring for her father. She had given up a good job and often was emotionally drained at the end of the day. She was very angry at the loss of the father she'd known, for they'd been very close.

Many people have talked with me about the dissension in their families. Family members would argue about the best care for the Alzheimer's patient. Some did not want to spend the money on their loved one's care while others argued that "Dad can't go to a nursing home; we promised him we'd handle everything for him."

One woman talked with me about feeling alone and isolated from her friends and normal routine. Her life wasn't hers any longer. Her uncle, whom she was caring for, wanted to stay up all night and sleep all day. He picked at his food and was incontinent. She felt increasingly angry at her situation.

John told me, "I am angry because my wife and I had planned to travel when I retired. I never thought my wife would get Alzheimer's—she's only 57. We saved all our lives for the future, and now this. She isn't my wife anymore. She was vibrant and smart and witty. Now all she wants to do is sleep. I feel so alone."

Another woman told me, "My sister was the caregiver for our mother and father; they both had Alzheimer's. My sister starved our mother to death and now she's doing the same thing to Dad. I've begged her to do right by our folks, but she just tells me to mind my own business. My sister controls the funds." This woman cried and said, "I lost my husband and am barely getting by myself, and I can't fight this case. I am so angry with my sister for mistreating our parents." I told her that her anger was justified in some respects. I told her to try to speak with a social worker, and that I'd pray for her.

Sometimes the loved one will "shadow" the caregiver, or follow them everywhere. This can make the caregiver angry as well. The Alzheimer's patient often can no longer remember how to perform the simplest tasks—climbing stairs, for example. They may not know how to move their feet from step to step, so they will follow the caregiver to watch what they do. The caregiver represents security for the person with Alzheimer's.

I had to try hard to not get angry with my mother when she would repeat the same thing over and over again. With training and discipline I managed to accept where my mother was for the moment, and eventually it no longer bothered me.

Sometimes the caregiver becomes angry because they cannot control the situation. Believe me, you will have no control over the behavior of an Alzheimer's patient. It helps if you tell yourself that it's the disease and not the person that's bothering you. Who really cares if the patient insists that the walls are green when they really are white? There is no right answer at this point.

Caregivers need to make the effort to take care of themselves as well as their patients. Otherwise they become tired and depressed, and then angry. Respite care and support groups can help with this situation. Sometimes a lack of training will lead to a lack of understanding, and also to anger. Exhaustion and lack of understanding can lead to abuse in some cases.

Abuse comes in many forms: verbal, physical, and emotional. The caregiver must always remember that the person they're caring for is no longer the same person; there is always a huge change in personality as the disease progresses. Oftentimes the patient him- or herself will become verbally abusive. Often a well-trained stranger can cope with an Alzheimer's patient better than a loved one can, because they have a bit of emotional distance in addition to extensive training.

Anger is a normal emotion. Good people get angry in difficult situations. Learn how to respond to your feelings of anger in a proper fashion. Think before you react.

Ultimately, my love for my mother helped me most of all in controlling my anger. She needed all the support I could give her, and she was my mom. Remembering that helped me through the worst times.

Listening and Learning About Other Caregivers' and Families' Situations

As I worked in the various nursing homes I realized how caregivers grieved over the loss of their loved ones to Alzheimer's. Two men told me their stories. Both had been married to their mates for many years. They were losing their soul mates, the women they'd shared their lives with, and were both beside themselves trying to figure out how to do the right thing for the ones they loved the most in the whole world.

Mr. C. had taken care of his wife for five years in their home. He spent every waking moment with her. He had to watch her communication skills declining and becoming very limited. She was losing weight and not eating. He never did much cooking before her illness and was struggling with figuring out how to make nutritious meals to help her sustain her weight. He felt very responsible for the person he loved so much. One day he decided to make meat loaf. He served the meal. His wife ate a couple of bites, then stopped eating and said,

"No." He pleaded with her to just eat a little more because he wanted her to stop losing weight. He started to cry. She stood up and said, "Now stop your crying—you are a grown man!" At that point he began to laugh. "And you are a grown woman. You should eat when and what you want to eat." While he always made sure meals were made, from that day forward, he never pushed her to eat at a certain time again.

After five years of being the caregiver, Mr. C. knew it was time to place his wife in a care facility. He felt so bad and wondered how he was going to tell her she was moving. He no longer could care for her himself. He took her clothes to the facility the night before because he didn't want her to feel bad. He wondered how she would feel about his putting her in a care facility. The next day he drove her to her new home. He asked the director if he should stay and have lunch with her. The director said, "She is not looking for you, so I would just go." His wife never asked to go home. She never realized that she was sick. She was content. He was very supportive of the care facility and his wife until her death. I witnessed his deep love for his wife. He was one of the most caring, kind people I have ever met in my life. I consider him an outstanding humanitarian for he has extended his love not only to his wife and family but also to countless people throughout his lifetime.

Mr. W.'s wife had knee surgery after she fell and broke her knee, and she had both of her knees replaced. She did not do her therapy at home as the doctor had instructed, so the doctor put her in a rehabilitation hospital. She could not remember to do the exercises in therapy. Mr. W. made excuses for his wife and covered for her. Finally he sent her to a neurologist and had her tested by a psychologist. The MRI showed that she was probably in the early stages of Alzheimer's. Mr. W. was in denial. He did take his wife to the doctor every six weeks. He felt a terrible amount of guilt. The two had retired and moved to Arizona. After consulting with his family he decided to return to Milwaukee, Wisconsin. He could not handle his wife and was very tired. He placed her in a care unit and took an apartment in an adjoining independent living unit so he could be close to her. Mr. W. sometimes became depressed because it was hard for him to watch his wife's decline. He had a good support system and stayed active, which helped him in his daily life. He too stayed very involved in his wife's care planning and came over for her meals. He was a very dedicated husband.

When Judy was planning to move her mom to a care facility, she thought it would be a good idea first to gather the family around to reminisce. The family meant well. They brought pictures and talked about the good old days. It was intended to be a happy send-off for Mable, but instead it alarmed and upset her. She was very worried about leaving her home, and having all the family there made her even more anxious and agitated.

One of the elderly ladies that I run errands for has a husband with Alzheimer's. She didn't pay attention to some of his ways at first. She just thought it was old age creeping up. For years Mr. R. took his car into the same shop for repairs and would leave it for the day. The repair man would drive him home and then return with the car at the end of the day. But one day, he took his car in and didn't come back home. His wife began to worry. At noon she called the repair shop and asked for Mr. R. The repair man said he had never showed up. She then panicked and called her son. Her son came over and finally Mr. R. returned. His wife said, "Where were you?" He said, "I don't remember. I did get help to get back home." Then the family took Mr. R. to the doctor and discovered he had Alzheimer's. Fortunately their daughter is a nurse. She and her mother went to classes and learned how to care for Mr. R. The entire family showed support and all pitched in to keep him independent as long as possible. Mrs. R. cared for him in their home for seven years. He was placed in a nursing care facility. The family continued to visit him and take him treats until his death. Mrs. R. shared with me that she recalls how as the disease began to affect him, Mr. R. would get mad while playing cards and walk off. In all of the years in card club he had never before become angry while playing cards. His anger was a result of not being able to follow the cards, and that was his way of covering up.

I recently met a lovely woman named Pearl who told me she was 94 years old. Her 74-

year-old daughter, (Pearl's only child) lived with her and was suffering from Alzheimer's. They have home health care right now, but Pearl worried about her daughter's future—there were no other family members to take over the caregiving when Pearl was gone. Theirs is an unusual situation, but devastating nonetheless.

Long Distance Caregiving

Many adult children live far from their parents. But there are still ways for them to remain involved with their parents' care. Their decisions are very important. I know a woman whose parents both suffer from Alzheimer's. She is a long-distance caregiver, who is very concerned about her parents. She uses her time wisely. She talked to their neighbors, friends, and relatives in hopes that they would share what they see about her parents.

If you are in this position it is best to make periodic visits. Make appointments with the physician, lawyer, and financial adviser when you visit. Do activities with your loved one such as going for a walk or listening to music.

Ask friends to visit your loved one at least once a week or for whatever time they can give. Even if the Alzheimer's patient does not remember the visit it still is important to visit. It helps for the moment. There are also people from religious or neighborhood groups that can help. Some religious organizations have volunteer outreach programs to help the elderly.

You may have to take time off from your job during crisis periods. You may consider looking into the Family and Medical Leave Act which allows a person to take leave for up to twelve weeks without pay, depending on the size of the company you work for.

Really think things through before you move your loved one from familiar surroundings. Often this may cause the person to become agitated and confused. Talk to your loved one's physician and social worker. If you move the person to your home you need to have 24-hour care and include the rest of the family living in the same household. You also need to get educated about how to deal with a person with Alzheimer's. Also, make sure you are financially capable of caring for your loved one.

Many families that are far from their loved one will send cards and little treats, and e-mail or telephone. You may be able to help the primary caregiver (with permission) by handling bills, filling out necessary papers, and learning about support services available in the caregiver's community. Above all it is important to keep communication lines open with all family members involved.

For More Information

- Write the U.S. Department of Health and Human Services, 2101 East Jefferson Street, Rockville, MD 20852.

- Children of Aging Parents
www.caps4caregivers.org.

- There is an Eldercare Locator, which is a free service to help you find local resources like adult day programs, respite care, elder abuse/protective agencies, Medicaid information, and transportation. Call (800) 677-1116.

- The local Area Agency on Aging (AAA) has services to help with long-distance caregiving. A home health care worker can be hired to help the person with bathing, toileting, preparing meals, and taking medication. Having an informal support system can help give the caregiver peace of mind.

Other Resources:

- The National Insurance Consumer Help Line, Washington, D.C. (800) 942-4242.

- American Association of Retired Persons (AARP), Washington, D.C. 1-888-687-2277.

- *Ambiguous Loss* by Pauline Boss, a book for caregivers to learn how to live with unresolved grief.

Chapter 4:

Skills the Caregiver Needs

Learning Caregiving Skills Through Observation and Experience

A social worker gave me a book and in simple words it told Mom the story about her memory loss. I read it with her as instructed by the social worker. Mom didn't understand everything I read, but she knew she was losing her memory. She lamented the loss of her independence. I had to be the bad guy and take away her car keys and car because she could no longer recognize common symbols, and she ran stop signs. Unfortunately, adult children have a very difficult time taking away the car keys. I felt I made the best decision; I could not live with myself if my mother hurt herself or anyone else.

Tips for Caring for an Alzheimer's Patient in Your Home

- Learn the person's habits.
- Get a daily routine and stick with it.
- Make activities a part of your daily routine and involve the person in them. (My mother loved housekeeping, so dusting and folding towels was a part of her routine.)
    - a. Preparing meals, cooking, eating.
    - b. Dusting, sweeping, and folding towels.
    - c. Bathing, shaving, and dressing.
- Focus on having fun.
- Don't force the person to achieve goals for the day.

- Live for the moment.
- Provide a safe and loving environment to meet the person's needs.
- Be thoughtful of the person's likes, dislikes, strengths, and abilities.
- Play upon the person's past interests.
- Prioritize—don't try to do everything when you are feeling overwhelmed.
- Learn as much as you can about Alzheimer's. The more you know, the better you can help yourself and your loved one. Especially learn about the Alzheimer's patient's past to be able to get into their own world and to better serve them.

Suggested Activities

Physical:	You can use a lightweight ball to play catch or exercise with music.
Social:	Have coffee with them or play cards. When we played together, my mom forgot some of the card game and confused two games. I went right along with it, and let her make up her own rules. She had fun for the moment. Playing cards the right way was less important than letting her enjoy the experience.
Intellectual:	I read to my mom. Others may enjoy working a crossword puzzle or looking at a colorful map of the United States to help them remember what state they are living in.
Spiritual:	Read a verse from their religious texts, pray, sing a spiritual song.
Creative:	Do a painting, color, or play a musical instrument.
Work-related:	If the patient is good at fixing something let him help.
Be Spontaneous:	Go for a ride with the person and the family or a friend.

They may enjoy going out for lunch. I would take Mom out for her favorite sandwich. My mom took pleasure in having her back scratched and her hair shampooed. Above all create an atmosphere where the person feels needed even if they just empty a waste basket. The happy patient most often will not become so readily anxious, irritable, or distracted. Some Alzheimer's patients cannot tolerate noises and will become frightened or agitated, while others love watching their favorite sports team. Some will like company and others will be totally unaware of the person visiting. Just go along with their moods.

The caregiver will keep his/her sanity by going with the flow. Activities generally lessen undesirable behavior such as wandering or agitation.

A good reference book is *Understanding Difficult Behavior* by Anne Robinson and Beth Spencer. The book is available from Eastern Michigan University, Ypsilanti, MI. You can order be calling (734) 487-2335 or fax (734) 487-0298 or on the internet at: www.emich.edu/public/Alzheimers. You can also call the southeastern Wisconsin Alzheimer's chapter at (414) 479-8800 and they will ship you a book.

What to Think About When Planning Activities

- The person: What do they like to do? The person may have a talent for or find pleasure in doing a particular activity. Does the person have any physical problems to hinder the activity?

- The activity: Do the activity as part of the person's daily routine, and have fun. Make the person feel needed. Adapt the activity to meet the person's skill level and needs. Think of the time of day for doing each activity (e.g., bathing and dressing in the morning). As the disease progresses, adapt to the situation.

- Your approach: Give support and simple, step-by-step directions. Work with the process, not toward the end product. Be flexible. If the person does it differently, don't get hung up on that—just fix it later. Compliment the person for their accomplishments. Take little breaks throughout the day.

- Some patients may require an afternoon nap or a short mid-morning nap. Don't let them sleep all day long with no activity in their daily routine or the person will become lethargic. Give him/her a sense of belonging, security, and appreciation for being there. Let him/her help by stirring the batter for a cake, or working on a card for a friend or family member. Be patient and take plenty of time to accomplish each task at the patient's pace. If the patient is not interested at the time, put the task away and try later. Time of day makes a big difference. Knowing the patient's mood swings during the day can make a big difference. Don't criticize or correct him. Help the person do the task as independently as possible. Encourage him/her to express themselves in a positive manner. You just don't know what they are thinking sometimes. If a person is acting out, try to do an activity to redirect them. Sometimes I found that just walking away from my mom when she became moody worked. It can be trial and error.

■ The environment: Be sure activities are safe. While Mabel was living in her own home on the farm, she was used to going out to get the mail every day at one o'clock. Now that Mabel is living with her daughter, Julie, it is difficult to do the same routine. The mail carrier comes late in the afternoon, and her daughter lives on a very busy street. It is not safe for Mabel to cross the road to get to the mailbox. Julie called the post office and got a post office box; now her husband picks up the mail and takes it home. They put up a special mailbox for Mabel by the house, and they make sure there is some mail for her so she can go out at one o'clock each day. That brings Mabel some pleasure in her daily routine and also she feels useful.

■ Make a plan for the day: morning (bathe, brush hair, brush teeth, dress, eat breakfast, do some chores together, have coffee, walk or exercise together); afternoon (make lunch, do dishes, do some gardening, watch a favorite TV show, take a nap); evening (prepare and eat dinner, clean up dishes, load dishwasher, reminisce, have a family dessert time). The main thing to remember is to include your loved one in family activities as much as possible or as the person will let you. Always offer them the chance to participate and feel needed, wanted, and special.

Be Flexible and Adaptable

My mom loved to pick tomatoes and raspberries. She also ate as many raspberries as she picked, but that was okay. She was having fun and she felt useful.

Yes, it takes extra work and effort to accommodate a loved one with Alzheimer's but it is worth it. It will save you some grief in the long run. If the person is a wanderer, rig up some type of bell on the doors for when they may roam out, or put up a fence around the yard and make sure the person wears a wander guard. When an Alzheimer's patient cannot recall familiar sounds or surroundings they may become frightened and very confused. Do help them so they feel comfortable in their surroundings. Have a smoke detector. It may save you and your family's lives. Help the person reminisce by looking through photo albums, listening to music, singing, looking through magazines related to their past hobbies, scrapbooks, or an old purse filled with memories. It helps the person create pleasures for the moment.

There will be a time in the last stages that the person may not be able to relate to any of these items. But even when my mom was nearing her death I still sang, prayed, and reminisced with her. I believe she could still hear me and there was still a part of her that could understand me. Your treatment of the Alzheimer's patient is so crucial for their comfort and dignity.

I took care of an Alzheimer's patient once who was close to her death. While I was praying with her the women held my hand very tightly. She told me in a lucid moment that her daughter had mistreated her terribly while she was living with her. She wanted to die to escape further abuse. I hugged her and she did not want to let go of me. I was very sad for this old woman. She died two weeks later and I still think of her. I hope she is now at peace with God at her side and that joy has entered her heart.

Incontinence and the Alzheimer's Patient

Incontinence is very common among the elderly, affecting twice as many men as women, especially for those over the age of 70, although it can begin as early as 60. It is especially common in Alzheimer's patients in the last stages of the disease.

My mother was incontinent in the later stages of Alzheimer's and had to wear disposable briefs. At first she requested to go to the bathroom every ten minutes. The doctor told us that what she had was defined as urge incontinence. The person that suffers with urge incontinence may have to get up several times a night and may occasionally wet the bed. This type of incontinence happens when the muscle that controls the flow of urine works in an abnormal fashion. As my mother's Alzheimer's progressed, so did her incontinence. She eventually had a total loss of bladder control—she was no longer even aware that she was urinating.

A person can become incontinent if the urethra is weakened. Sometimes surgery can correct the problem, but there is a risk of nerve damage. Stress can also cause minor incontinence, causing some leaking. Sneezing, laughing, and coughing can also result in some leakage. Incontinence can also be a side effect of diabetes. Certain medications can also cause some incontinence—check with your doctor if you are taking medicine, especially antidepressants or heart medication—and check with your doctor if you develop incontinence, to rule out any underlying medical causes.

The elderly are very susceptible to urinary tract infections (UTIs). UTIs can be treated with medications, but may require hospitalization, as the elderly can become quite ill and weak with a serious UTI. Any signs of a UTI should immediately be brought to the attention of a doctor.

Incontinence can be embarrassing and can make the patient feel depressed and isolated. They may withdraw and refuse to socialize. No one should need to feel ashamed of being incontinent. The caregiver should deal with the depression and isolation immediately.

While I was working in a care facility during my training days, an Alzheimer's patient went into the facility's beauty parlor. She thought that the beauty parlor was the bathroom. She pulled down her pants and urinated and defecated on the chair. I helped the caretaker clean up the lady and the beauty parlor. That was the first and last time that type of incident happened because we worked on an incontinence maintenance schedule for her, following her habits to better meet her needs. The patient never realized what she'd done, and we, of course, never reprimanded her. These things can happen with an Alzheimer's patient, whether in a care facility or at home.

A caregiver at home should practice incontinence management by monitoring the patient's bathroom needs and habits. The caregiver must act in the best interest of the patient, and should not appear overly anxious about the bouts of incontinence. If the patient wears disposable briefs, check them periodically, especially before and after meals and at bedtime, to make sure the patient stays dry. Remember that the Alzheimer's patient may not realize that they've become wet. Try to keep them clean and dry to prevent rashes and foul odors. Above all, the caregiver must stay calm, never shaming or scolding the patient who's had an accident. The caregiver should take a few deep breaths if they become frustrated or angry.

Your local drugstore or grocery store carries many styles of disposable undergarments.

It can be trial and error to find the right undergarment for your loved one. Some of these disposable briefs are fastened with buttons, others with Velcro. Buttons may be difficult to manage for patients with arthritis in their hands. On the other hand, a patient who does not want to wear the briefs may be able to get out of the Velcro garments more easily than those that are fastened with buttons. Above all, make sure that the disposable briefs fit the patient comfortably and do not bind.

For more information call the National Kidney Foundation at (800) 622-9010, write them at 30 East 33rd Street, New York, NY 10016, or check out their website, www.kidney.org and also the National Association for Continence at (800) 252-3337 or (800) BLADDER (Spartanburg, SC).

Getting Help in Your Home as Alzheimer's Progresses

You may want some assistance so you, the caregiver, can get away. A companion can come in and play cards or relieve you for just an hour or two during the day. The friend can do some grocery shopping, help with laundry and meal preparation. There are trained home care aides that can come in and assist with bathing and grooming, hair and nail care, toileting, and dressing. There are therapeutic services and dietitian consultations, pharmacy and medical supply services that can help take the burden from you.

Of course, payment depends on the amount of services rendered for you in your home. You can set up payment plans—also, private insurance or Medicare may cover some of the cost. When someone has enough money to pay on their own, they generally get better care. Check with your local doctor and insurance company to make sure who pays the bill. Make sure that any home health care service you use is accredited. It may also help if the agency is nonprofit. In my experience I have found that the for-profit home care agency is more interested in just making a dollar while the nonprofit agency is sincere and wants to help the elderly. In all fairness, there may be many for-profit agencies that provide wonderful care. You will get superior service if you find people with endless compassion and are true advocates for their patients.

Caregiver Stress

One mistake caregivers make is they don't take care of themselves. As a result they become agitated and very stressed out. Not only do you hurt yourself but also you hurt the person for whom you are caring. The caregiver must be very aware of the ten signs of caregiver stress in order to act in the proper manner.

1. Denial. "Dad's not so forgetful after all; I can leave him home while I do the grocery shopping."
2. Anger. "Why does he keep repeating so often? I told him four times already. Why does he have to be such a burden on me? I am so angry that I have to be responsible for him."
3. Social withdrawal. "I can't go to the neighbor's for coffee anymore. I don't care about socializing any longer. I am burdened with my mom."
4. Anxiety. The caregiver worries about what tomorrow may bring. "Dad just wandered away yesterday and I spent two hours frantically looking for him. Now what will happen today? Will he do that again?"
5. Depression. "Life just isn't worth living anymore. I don't care about anything. I am so overwhelmed and down."
6. Exhaustion. "I am too tired to do anything anymore. I can't get my work accomplished."
7. Sleeplessness. "I stay awake night after night worrying about my Dad wandering somewhere." Sometimes, doctors can give patients who wander something to get them to sleep at night and stay up during the day.
8. Irritability. The caregiver becomes irritable with the most trivial thing, taking it out on the patient. This is where abuse could take place, because the caregiver is at his/her wits' end. "Just everyone go away and leave me alone!" The caregiver has no peace of mind.
9. Lack of concentration. "I can't think any longer to get my work done. My thought process just is not in order. Oh no! I just missed my doctor's appointment yesterday. I waited two months to get in to that doctor. Now I'll have to reschedule. Anyhow I couldn't go yesterday I was too busy taking care of my dad."
10. Health problems. The caregiver gets up every morning feeling sick to their stomach; their mental health begins to suffer.

The family is deeply affected when their loved one has Alzheimer's. Everyone reacts differently and the disease can break up a family. This, in itself, is very sad and disheartening.

Here are some suggestions for a family dealing with Alzheimer's—become educated; stay on the same page with every family member; be realistic; involve all family members; get involved with the Alzheimer's Association; remember your loved one; visit and help as much as possible; be supportive and listen; find a support group to help you get through difficult times.

Many people for whom placing a parent in a care facility is unthinkable bring them into their own homes without fully realizing what caring for an Alzheimer's patient entails. Especially as the disease progresses, it is a 24-hour-a-day job. It is not enough to give them a room, clothing, and meals, and expect them to quietly watch TV. The person may become agitated by noisy grandchildren, or may wander and get lost, or may become combative or sexually aggressive. It is best to give the person adequate stimulation and the opportunity to socialize with people of their own age. Adult day care centers have many activities tailored for Alzheimer's patients.

Isolation Issues for Both the Patient and the Caregiver

People with Alzheimer's often battle loneliness and depression. In many cases, it is because the patient may have outlived most of their family and friends. Other times, family and friends don't visit because they too are in poor health, or they live far away, or simply because they don't know what to say to the person. It is painful for them to see the way the disease has changed the person they once knew. Even telephone calls become difficult for the patient as the disease progresses and they grow increasingly incoherent. If a patient becomes comatose, family finds it especially difficult to continue to visit. They think, "That isn't the person I knew, and she doesn't know me any longer. What is the use of visiting?" It isn't only that they don't think it's helpful to the person, it is also because it's very painful for them. They fear becoming like the patient themselves someday. But I believe visiting the sick is a work of mercy and a charitable act.

When my mother and aunt were ill, I just knew that somehow visiting them was the right thing to do. When I couldn't do anything else, I could just hold their hands. It was just good to be there for them and honor them. They had been there for me earlier in my life; this was the time they needed me to be there for them.

The disease takes a toll on the patient, but it also takes a toll on the caregiver. Caregivers can become depressed and isolated too, and they need to make it a priority to take time for themselves and ask for help when they need it. Their entire world may revolve around their loved one and the illness, but without some breaks from the daily routine and stress a person will eventually burn out or crack under the pressure. It's easy to think, "I can't take time for a bridge game, or exercise—I'll never get everything done!" But you need your breaks. Trust me, I know. Because I took the time I needed for myself, I was able to remain calm and very patient with my mother. Caregivers need to remember not to neglect other family relationships; spouses and children need attention, too.

I was doing a book signing recently in Iowa, and a young boy about ten years old came up to me with his mom. "What are you selling?" he asked. I told him I was selling my book *Picnics: Catering on the Move* in honor of my mother because I lost her to Alzheimer's and then to death. "My great-grandmother has that awful disease," said the boy. "She no longer knows me."

"How do you feel about that?" I asked him.

"Very sad," he said.

I asked him if he'd ever asked the kids in his class if they had a favorite relative with the disease. He said, "No."

"Perhaps you can become a friend to someone who is also feeling sad about the loss of someone to this disease," I suggested. His mom said she thought that sounded like a good idea. "I am your friend," I told him, "and I know how you are feeling." He gave me a hug and said thank you. It was a heartfelt moment for both of us.

Breaks for the Caregiver

Very often an Alzheimer's patient will become very possessive of their caregiver. They will follow someone closely. The Alzheimer's patient can become very demanding and upset if they cannot see the caregiver.

Almost every caregiver I have spoken with has lost patience with their loved one at some point because they were spending every waking moment with that person. If the patient confuses day and night, and the caregiver is unable to get enough sleep, it becomes even harder. Remember, if you don't take care of yourself, you can't take care of anyone else. Seek help when you need it. Trying to do everything on your own will only lead to frustration and feelings of isolation and helplessness. I can't stress enough, it can be a cause of caregivers' abusing or neglecting Alzheimer's patients.

Without the support system I relied on, I couldn't have kept my sanity. I avoided feeling isolated and lonely because I used all the resources I could find to help me better understand my mother's condition.

Reaching out helps in many ways. My deepest pain of losing my mother—twice—has been healed because I have reached out to others and surrounded myself with wonderful people in my life that genuinely care. That and my faith have carried me through the most difficult times. And though I didn't seek it, the pain in my life has brought much fruit. My dad always told me if you have no pain in life, you have no gain, and in my case he was correct.

Testing for Alzheimer's

- ■ Determine their daily habits and their current mental status.
- ■ Get a mental status evaluation. I took my mother to the hospital for this test, that lasted two hours.
- ■ Get a physical examination. Be sure to get blood pressure, nutritional status, and pulse checked. I had Mom take a CAT scan for she had had a series of mini-strokes which affected her short-term memory.
- ■ Get a neurologist to examine and evaluate the person closely. There may

be a brain tumor causing memory impairment instead of Alzheimer's. Make sure the physician checks out the following items: coordination, speech and sensation, eye movement, muscle tone, and strength.

■ Get a series of laboratory tests. Through these tests the physician can rule out other diseases. The doctor can order an EEG (electro-encephalogram). This will reveal any abnormal brain wave activity. The CT (computerized tomography) scan takes X-ray images of the brain. This shows evidence of tumors, strokes, and blood clots. The MRI (magnetic resonance imaging) is a brain-imaging technique used for finding out information about the brain. The PET (positron emission tomography) shows how different areas of the brain respond when the person is asked to perform different activities such as exercising or talking. SPECT (single proton emission computed tomography) reveals how blood is flowing to the brain.

■ Get psychiatric, psychological, and other evaluations. I took my mom through several tests and a psychological evaluation with a nurse and a senior health social worker. When I took Mom for her testing I made sure she had her glasses along. She refused to wear her hearing aids. I might add it is very difficult to force someone to wear their hearing aids if they refuse. (Do not fight with them on the issue; it just makes for a difficult situation.) My mom was physically healthy and did not take any medications at the time. Be sure you have his/her social security number, medical records, insurance number, and information to be prepared for the exam. The tests definitely showed me that Mom had poor judgment, memory impairment, and language problems that prevented her from functioning independently on a day-to-day basis. After going through all the tests, there was no doubt in my mind that my mom had Alzheimer's. At that point it meant that there was going to be a lot of family decision-making. I kept in touch with the professionals.

Help for Wanderers

If your loved one is a wanderer you may need to order a safe return bracelet. To learn more about the Safe Return program call your local chapter of the Alzheimer's Association.

The safe return identification bracelet enables anyone who finds the person with

Alzheimer's to get the patient home safely. You fill out a form with information about the person with Alzheimer's and tell whom to contact if the person is found.

Wandering and Agitation

One woman thought she could lock her mom safely in her home and run to the store, and her mom would be safe alone. Upon returning from the grocery store she saw that her mom was missing. It was in the dead of winter and ten degrees below zero. After two days of searching the search team found her mom in a nearby field frozen to death. Please believe me: it is a 24-hour-a-day job to care for a loved one with this disease.

My mom never wandered from the group home. Some residents had to be watched constantly because they would wander away. It was a safety issue if the wanderer got away.

I recall taking Mom for lunch one time. To my surprise she wanted pizza. She never ate pizza. I stayed with her in line while we ordered pizza. We sat down and waited for our number to be called. When I went up to get the pizza, she slipped away in the crowd. I was frantic because we were in a shopping center. I alerted security and we searched until we found her. She was sitting on a shopping center bench crying. I threw my arms around her and praised God for her safety. She said, "Why did you leave me?" I was speechless. I never again let her out of my sight nor did I ever take her to a shopping center again. While I had only left my mom for a very short time, I understood the consequences of wandering all too well with this episode.

I first learned about agitation through observation of my mother's behavior. Mom would pace and get impatient and say "let's go" repeatedly. I would ask her where she would like to go. I would walk with her and hold her hand. Then I learned to mirror her by saying, "So you want to go." "Yes," she'd reply. I then was not questioning her but mirroring her thoughts and recognizing her feelings. Sometimes I got her a cup of decaf coffee (her favorite drink) and would speak softly to her to help her calm down.

The hardest part for me was watching my mother go backwards with this degenerative mental disease. It's easy to understand a child's conduct. However, we know the child will someday grow up. But my mom and my aunt had already grown up and raised families. Both lived full adult lives. Now in my mind both were going backwards and fading into the twilight. Mom's behavior in particular was not always acceptable. It was not a pretty sight to see her go backwards. I began to realize that I had to accept this major change in my mother. I also learned coping skills from the classes I took, and learned that as the brain cells died she would become increasingly mentally incapacitated.

Mom had behavior disturbances. Her personality changed greatly and sometimes she became combative. Mom had difficulty in recalling names and eventually she could not write.

Due to Mom's mental status she could not remember to eat. When I first discovered her problem she had rotten food in her refrigerator. I replaced the food, but that did not help. Fortunately, I asked for help and was able to take her out of her home and bring her to a safe place.

One woman bought food for her mother, but the woman did not know enough to prepare the food, or even eat for that matter. Actually, she thought she had already eaten. She died of starvation.

Another gentleman would not believe that his mother had Alzheimer's. (As I have mentioned elsewhere, denial is very common among adult children.) He took his mother to his home and left, thinking there was nothing wrong. He returned to find his house burned down and his mother dead.

Other Common Behaviors

The Alzheimer's patient's complete disconnection from reality can create extremely frustrating situations for caregivers.

In one case, Jimmy a man who had been diagnosed with the disease, had been doing fairly well in the care of his daughter and other supportive family members. In the middle of the night, Jimmy decided he wanted to go swimming in the old swimming hole. He imagined that the toilet was the swimming hole, and tried climbing into it. His daughter had heard him and came looking for him, but he became agitated and said, "I'm going swimming—go away." Her efforts to reason with him and to get him out of the toilet only made him more adamant. Finally, she called the doctor, an old family friend, to come over. He gave Jimmy a shot of muscle relaxant, and they were able to extract his foot from the toilet.

In another case, Dan a retired funeral home director with Alzheimer's, found the keys his family had hidden away and drove away in the funeral home hearse. When they discovered he was gone, the family panicked, called police, and began a frantic search for him.

A neighbor found him at the cemetery, talking earnestly at his wife's grave. When the neighbor tried to get him to return home, Dan was irritated. "I'm talking to Ana now. Don't interrupt me!" The neighbor told him, "I'm sorry I interrupted you, Dan, but we really need you back at the funeral home. Mr. Big's wife has died, and he needs you to come right away. He really trusts you and knows you'll take care of him. I can bring you back later to talk to Ana." This way, he was able to persuade Dan to come back with him. He didn't ask, "What are you doing here? What is wrong with you? You can't drive anymore!" That would only have served to agitate Dan and upset them both.

While I was working in a care facility, I met a man who'd grown up on a farm. He loved to tell me about his horses. One day he told me his horse was waiting for him downstairs and we must go down to get it. I engaged him in conversation about the horse, asking various questions. "What color is your horse?"

"It's white."

"Well, I just came in a minute ago, and I did see a beautiful black horse, but not a white one. Yours must be coming later. Come on with me to the music room and we can sing for a while." He came with me.

Another time in a facility, a man stripped off all his clothes. Caregivers calmly came and redressed him, took him for a walk, and then several of us sang with him to soothe and redirect him. In another case, I saw a caregiver following a lady around as she walked on her tiptoes. She preferred to eat on the run. It took two people to feed her, so her family members would come at lunch to help. She was in constant motion, and caring for her was an exhausting task.

Mom could not understand distance. While she was 200 miles away from home she asked me to go home and look in her cupboard for her favorite date bread recipe. I would say, okay, Mom. I can do that for you. I already had her recipe and so the next day I would bring it to her. Of course, she did not even remember asking me to get the recipe.

When my mother became combative, which she did whenever she was afraid or imagined something was wrong, I would distract her by throwing my arms around her and saying, "I love you! You have such pretty blue eyes. Let me see those beautiful, smiling, blue eyes!" That would slow her down. Then she would giggle, and things would be okay. Other times, I would just walk away, leave her alone, and count to ten. I would then go back, and she'd be fine.

Sexual aggression is another common problem, but there are medications available to address this. This needs to be worked out with a doctor who is familiar with treating Alzheimer's patients. I firmly believe that a person shouldn't be drugged to the point that they cannot function and participate in activities.

Keep in mind that the patients never remember their actions. It is best not to bring the subject up again. Just take whatever reasonable measures necessary to prevent the situation again, if possible, such as making sure car keys are not within reach. In care facilities, electronic wander guards are placed on the ankles of patients who are inclined to wander. The device triggers an alarm if the person tries to leave the facility. One man I met in a support group had a loud horn installed that sounded when the front door opened so he would know if his mother opened it. He also fenced in the backyard with a latch on the gate that was difficult to open and out of her reach.

Communicating

language to accent the positive. Body language is a nonverbal

mother loved attention and she loved to be loved. If I held my

d and give me a hug. I don't really know of any human being that

howing my love to my mother helped me get through some of

When working in care facilities, I never walked up behind a patient because I did not want to scare them. I always talked to the person where they could see me. I used direct eye contact. I learned to always strive to make the person feel warm and relaxed whenever possible. I did not use jerky movements and did not hurry my mother or aunt. I went with their pace. I remember witnessing a family member saying something harsh about a patient in her presence. The patient cried and felt very badly. Never speak in front of the patient in any derogatory manner. You never know how much a person can comprehend. Some patients have selective hearing—they only hear what they want to hear. In addition, sometimes when you speak to the Alzheimer's patient they do not understand what you are saying to them. My aunt did a lot of smiling but often did not know what we were asking or saying. She did not know how to respond. Nevertheless she was always pleasant and happy. Understanding the Alzheimer's patient's word substitution and communication is very important. A patient may say no when they mean yes. The caregiver must be tuned in to understand and respond in an appropriate manner. I think of my aunt, Gene, often. She would speak and make no sense. She repeated everything over and over. It alarmed the family, which led to the discovery of Alzheimer's.

As my mom and aunt lost mental status both failed to recognize sensory stimuli. Giving cues helped to accomplish a task or assist the memory somewhat in the beginning of the disease. A landmark or image on the door may help the resident recognize his/her room. I expected nothing fantastic from my mom and aunt. I would rejoice when a breakthrough was accomplished.

Fears and Delusions

It is not uncommon for a patient to decline a bath. My mother had a lot of fears about being bathed. I had to walk away and go back to getting her bathed a little later. Eventually, she would accept the bath. Having her hair and nails done often relieved stress and made her feel good.

At times, Mom would have problems with slurred speech and sometimes the words would not come out right. She would get very upset with herself. This would occur especially if she was overly anxious or tired.

Some caregivers have expressed shock when a patient becomes combative and uses profanity. I must admit I was shocked too the first time my mom used that language. She never swore in her life. I had to recognize it was just part of the disease.

At an Alzheimer's caregivers support group meeting, some family caregivers complained of their loved one accusing them of stealing their money. It is a form of delusion. The person cannot reason and understand evidence.

I remember getting a call from the banker in our hometown. The banker stated that my mother came into the bank and made quite a scene. She was bouncing checks and accused the banker of stealing her money. I closed down the account and took the checkbook away so this would not happen again. The banker was grateful, for he felt badly about what was happening to my mother. He could relate because his father also had Alzheimer's.

Some patients have hallucinations. They insist they see, hear, or feel something that is not there. One of my friend's husband was a meek, quiet man and very religious. When his Alzheimer's disease progressed he became hypersexually agitated and exhibited inappropriate sexual behavior.

My neighbor's cousin from Indiana had a big farm. He plowed his land for years. In fact, he grew up on that farm. One day he came in and said to his wife, "I can't find the tractor to get my work done." She said, "It is sitting right outside." He disagreed. He was only 57 at the time.

Failure to Recognize Family and Friends

I found it very difficult to cope with the Alzheimer's patient's inability to recognize family and friends and even herself. I worked very hard at accepting that my aunt no longer knew me. Sometimes my mom would recognize me and other times not.

I remember doing a hat show at a facility. Many of the caregivers brought in fancy hats and let the residents pose with the hats. I had a mirror for them to see how they looked. Some did not even recognize their own faces. I said, "That is you." Some said, in a perplexed voice, "Me?" I replied, "Yes, you." I continued by passing the mirror around and saying how pretty they looked with their hats. The residents enjoyed this experience.

As my mom's disease progressed she often did not remember me. I went to the doctor's office to be with her for an appointment. I said, "Hi Mom."

"Who are you?" she asked.

"I am your daughter, Pat," I responded.

"I don't have a daughter, Pat. My daughter Pat is dead."

My heart sank. Because I was working with Alzheimer's patients at the time, I began to help jog her memory by talking about the big tomatoes we planted together and all the pretty roses she grew over the years. Finally she said, "You really are alive. You are my daughter." She hugged me and began to cry. "I thought you were dead." I took her to the bathroom upon her request and she asked, "Where have you been? I am all alone!" Of course I assured her, "Mom, I am here and I love you with my whole heart and soul." After the doctor's appointment I took her out for lunch and she would not let me out of her sight. She was confused at the doctor's office and the doctor had to help her when she became combative. She was out of her environment and felt very threatened.

In a facility where I work weekly, one of the gentlemen is in a geri chair. His right eye is shut permanently, but he can track me with his left eye. While I was playing "Let Me Call You Sweetheart," he put his hands up to dance. He use to be a good dancer and always loved music. I felt good about communicating with him through my music.

In the early 1960s, when I was 19 years old, I worked at a nursing home. Nursing homes were different back then. One 89-year-old resident would call out for his mother and ask why she would not visit him. I would hold his hand and say your mom is probably busy doing chores, but she has not forgotten you. I would continue to hold his hand and talk gently to him and try to make him feel good. The head nurse was a retired army nurse. She had a very brusque bedside manner. She would say, "That is not true; your mother is dead." She also was very hard on the patients. I hated to watch her unkind treatment.

Working with My Aunt and Mother
Taught Me How to Help Others

My mother, in her second stage of Alzheimer's, would sit with me for an hour at a time and help me sort buttons. I would get her a needle with thread and she strung all the sorted buttons of the same colors, size, and texture. It kept her busy. She felt needed and useful. I still have some of those buttons in my button box today. It is a memory of her, and I do not have the heart to use those buttons. It was a team project with my mother that I cherish. Both Mom and I were button collectors. (Note: Very small buttons are very difficult for residents to pick up. Be sure that residents who put everything in their mouths do not participate in this activity without extra close supervision or not at all.)

My Aunt Gene was in the third stage of Alzheimer's. She was easy to visit. While she did not know me, she enjoyed the attention. She especially loved to look at cooking magazines and feel soft fabrics. Aunt Gene had been a great cook in her younger days. She also sewed her own clothes. I would sit next to Aunt Gene as we looked through the pretty pictures of food and feel the brightly colored fabrics. When it was time to go I would say "Goodbye, Aunt Gene," as I kissed her cheek and hugged her. Aunt Gene would say, "I don't know you, but you are a nice lady."

My aunt and uncle were married for over 60 years. My uncle grieved so when he lost my aunt to Alzheimer's. Fortunately for her she did not realize when her husband died for she no longer knew him. The family took her to the funeral. She would not grieve over the loss of her lifelong partner she no longer remembered. Accepting this emotional loss is heart wrenching to families and friends. I know how much I have grieved over losing my mother first to Alzheimer's and then to death. It is a long goodbye. I recite this saying to help me get comfort when I am feeling sad:

> Like the ocean comes in waves
> Only to recede
> And come yet again
> But with it comes healing,
> Memories wash ashore and are bathed by the golden sun.
> Grab hold of those memories and let them fill the emptiness.
> May they bring you peace.

(Author unknown)

Boxes of Memories

I began to realize that Alzheimer's patients are truly in their own little world. The trick is to get into their world to share and love them and accept them at the present stage for their moment. Expect nothing and you will receive little perks and beautiful surprises. Since I worked with my loved ones sorting buttons and feeling fabrics, I thought this was an activity I could put together for other residents. Families can also participate in these types of activities. I thought of Aunt Gene liking all those pretty pictures of food. I got a high-functioning resident to clip pictures of foods with vivid colors. She also put together pictures in photo albums of vacations, sports, families, and other holiday themes. There are many forgotten folks in care facilities. This was a great tool for volunteers to use on a one-on-one visit.

From my experiences with my mom and aunt I decided to try putting together a kit made up of various fabrics so the residents with Alzheimer's could feel them. I also put together a box of buttons to sort. I had a box of socks to sort, nuts in a shell, different size pastas to match in a box. I also made up a board with the names of the pastas and pasted a sample of each by the name. Keep in mind as the disease progresses the resident will not be able to read and some will not be able to distinguish sizes. If the resident just recognizes one size or object, it is a plus.

As I watched my aunt feel the fabrics I found it helped her become more stimulated and enhanced her sensory skills. I also learned through my experiences that the more you know about the person and their daily living habits of the past the more you can serve the resident with love.

I worked with families to put together shoe boxes of items to help residents recall memories of their past. Families were very cooperative and gathered items that they also could use while visiting with their loved ones. So often I would hear families say "I don't know what to say or do when I visit Mom or Dad." The memory box is a very good one-on-one tool. One daughter made up a box with her mom's purse. Inside of the purse was her mom's wallet with a picture of her cat with her mother. Also there was a piece of fur in the same color as her mom's cat. The resident enjoyed the touch of the fur. It reminded her of her cat. There were other pictures in the wallet. Her mother always carried her purse everywhere. She was a social butterfly. This purse was a tool to help her mom think of the old times when she drove all over and went out to lunch with her friends and family. This made Mom happy for the moment.

Another family put together pictures and small antiques because the resident had run an antique shop in her younger days. Other sample boxes had baseball, fishing, and hunting themes. These served some of the male population. Some of the ladies also liked baseball and fishing. Each box fit the past interest of the individual resident.

I also brought in my seashell and rock collections for residents to sort by size. The colors also attracted the residents. I saved different size cans with labels and colorful bowls for residents to sort and nestle.

As I worked with third and fourth stage Alzheimer's patients, I saw that many could not recognize colors. They do appreciate bright colors such as red but could not tell me the name of the color. This is an example of visual agnosia. My aunt's face would become very bright when she saw vivid colors.

Some patients cannot recognize objects by feel. I showed flowers to one resident. She had been a gardener in her younger years. To the staff's surprise she named each of the flowers. Another resident put her hand in the sock filled with sugar. She said "sugar." She had been a baker at a school for 35 years. However, she could no longer recognize the Christmas tree on the sock.

For an art project I cut a colorful plastic placemat into rectangular shapes $2x2^1/_2$ inches. We sorted buttons as a group to fit on the rectangular shape. The residents could feel the textures and see the colors. Then we glued the buttons to the front of the placemat pieces, and a pin on the back. Each resident received a pin. All of these suggestions have worked for me in nursing homes and home settings. It just takes time to organize the kits. In my mom's case it helped her retain some recognition of sizes of objects. She liked helping me. So many residents feel useless. Mom also used her sensory skills with the sorting exercise.

Another thing I did with Mom was to take her for a drive sometimes around my neighborhood in southern Wisconsin. There are many church steeples in the area. We would count the steeples and notice the shapes and crosses. Mom had very good eyesight for her age. She had fun finding the steeples. It was a little awareness game I played with her while driving around town and in the country. On one of our rides we drove to the western part of the state in late March. It was 70 degrees and sunny. Mom always liked to ride in the car. Her friend had grown up in a little town in the area; she had always talked about the beautiful scenery in that part of the state. Mom got very excited when she saw the bluffs and the rock formations.

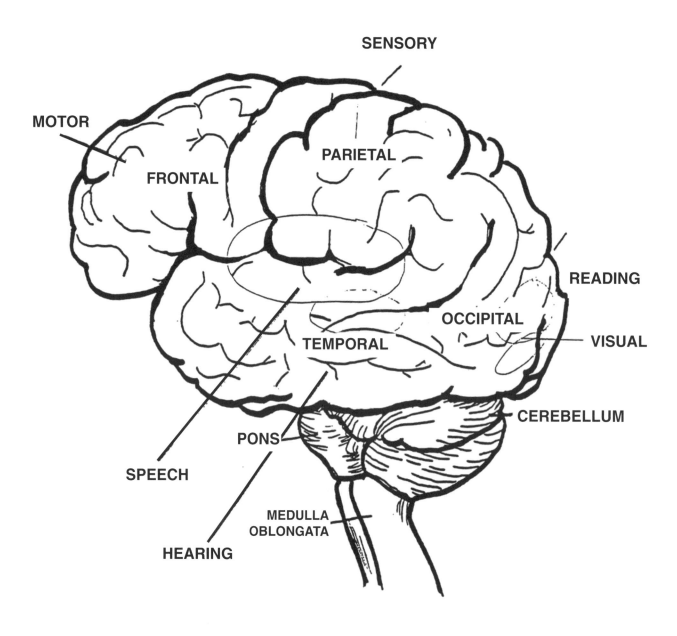

She said, "Oh, it is just beautiful!"

I went home that night and began to think about the sensory system. I decided to study about sensory integration. So I began my search for answers that I could apply to help other residents.

Sensory Integration

Every person is born with the chance to organize from their sensory system: vision, proprioception (the ability to receive stimuli from within the muscles, joints, and tendons), hearing, touch, smell, and taste. The sensory input must be integrated. If the brain does not process sensory information properly, the patient can experience sensory overload or deprivation. Sensory integration gives the person the ability to organize knowledge that we process. This process lets the person manage their own being within the environment.

For example, when all five senses work it gives the person a far greater chance to function at a higher level than with input from only one or two senses. A person may smell a scent that reminds him or her of a past experience. The smell probably stimulated the memory. In reality the scent was not the focal point of the actual experience, but it acted as a trigger. When the developmental process has been changed in any manner, persons do not have the sensory capability to react to their environment. Individuals experiencing sensory losses or loss of memory can rely on the sensory system to respond to their environment. They also can remember past events but cannot remember what they just ate. They also can reply to learned responses. The sensory integrative approach is used to increase or improve the brain's ability to learn to do things, but does not teach specific or basic skills.

A person with Alzheimer's needs ongoing sensory stimulation to live a good quality of life. The caregiver must be ready to take on these challenges with a good attitude and invent creative ways to accomplish this task.

A baby who lacks human touch and love develops a condition called "failure to thrive." This can easily threaten the survival of the baby. This same idea can be applied to the elderly population. They need hugs, love, and a basic level of sensory stimulation to sustain life.

There are four types of stimulation: sensory, social, emotional, and cognitive. In the case of an Alzheimer's patient, cognitive stimulation diminishes with each stage. It is crucial to provide stimulation through daily activity, environment, and one-on-one interactions. Remember that the emotions are always important in the life of the Alzheimer's patient. Respond to and treat the Alzheimer's patient the way you yourself would want to be treated. In fact this is a good rule to apply to every person you meet.

In a nursing home setting, a care plan should be in place to help the resident meet their stimulation needs. It is a crucial task for the Alzheimer's resident to continue to sustain life with dignity. When my mother was first placed in a care facility at her second stage of Alzheimer's, I always had something planned to help stimulate her. Even though she had memory loss she knew that sometime during the day I would be there to do activities with her.

One of the advantages of placing a loved one in an excellent care facility is the daily activities to stimulate the resident. Remember that as a family member, you need to be an advocate for your loved one. Be present often at the facility. Visit unannounced and at different times of the day. Stay involved in the sensory care plan for your loved one as well as their general health care plan. Be there and your loved one will get good care. I know this from my experience with my mother and working in care facilities. The squeaky wheel always gets the grease.

Care of an Alzheimer's patient in a family's home can be more difficult if the caregiver has a family to care for, not to mention a full-time job outside the home. If the patient is combative or a wanderer it can wear on the caregiver and family. The caregiver might have a tendency, out of frustration, to put the patient in a room in front of a TV. They will close the door and let them sleep. But this lack of stimulation is devastating.

If an Alzheimer's patient is poorly treated by a caregiver, the patient will die inside. It takes a caregiver who is willing to set aside their needs to meet the needs of the person in their care. There must be a deep feeling of love and responsibility.

Though they are strangers to the patients when they first arrive, caregivers in a facility often become very close to the residents. They form a bond and fill their hearts with love and concern for the residents.

Do whatever is possible within the patient's limitations to increase the level of awareness and alertness. Prevent sensory deprivation. With each individual use the senses to get them to respond to stimuli.

The Ten Deficits in Sensory Integration

1. Lack of sight discrimination (the inability to visually locate an object when asked).
2. Poor balance and poor body posture.
3. Attention deficit (can pay attention only a short time).
4. Lack of tactile discrimination (the inability to identify an object by touch).
5. Agitated.
6. Diminished visual comprehension (the inability to understand what they see).
8. Diminished tactile comprehension.
7. Poor judgment skills.
9. Easily distracted.
10. Irritable.

Goals of a Sensory Integration Focus

1. Use a social setting to hold or improve their physical, social, emotional, and cognitive functional abilities.
2. Even though members of a group may be at different cognitive levels, try to make every member comfortable and happy.
3. Expand their attention spans.
4. Develop their tolerance levels to physical cues.
5. Repeat work daily if possible with fine and large motor skills.
6. Increase their ability to interact with others.

7. Increase their ability to retain the maximum amount of physical and social jobs.

Note: *One of the problems in many of the care facilities is that everything is done for the patients. Try to keep each person as independent as possible for as long as possible.*

The Purpose of the Therapeutic Program

■ Get the residents in a group and have them rotate their heads and shoulders to increase flexibility.

■ Create activities that use the hands and fingers. This movement allows the brain to open up to new reception of knowledge.

Examples of Therapeutic Program activities:

■ Shaking jingle bells while keeping beat to the music during music therapy.

■ Waving flags to move muscles in the arms.

■ Clapping during a music program.

■ Hand massages.

■ Painting.

■ Stringing Cheerios.

■ Hand puppets.

■ Hand holding.

■ Games using the fingers and hands.

■ Activities involving different textures.

■ Activities involving use of scents.

Provide Body Awareness experiences:

■ Use marbles in sand in a shoe box for foot and hand massage.

■ File and paint nails.

■ Use paint rollers in art class. (This activity moves the left arm across to the right and vice versa. Thus this activity crosses the mid-line of brain hemispheres. This helps to strengthen both hemispheres, giving the resident a better chance to have a greater repertoire for responsiveness.) Encourage body movements like leaning forward or leaning back.

Group ideas:

■ Songs such as "If you are happy and you know it, clap your hands," and games such as "Simon Says." The activity director may help the resident touch the resident's hands to identify the body part.

Pet/baby therapy:

- Let the resident hold a pet in his/her lap and stroke the animal's fur.
- Rocking and holding a baby or baby doll.

While visiting my mother one day, I watched her rocking the nurse's ten-month-old baby. He was fussy, and she rocked him until he stopped crying. She enjoyed that time and bragged about how he stopped crying when she rocked him. When I travel to facilities I watch women hold baby dolls. I asked one lady how her baby was doing. She said, "I had a rough night last night. The baby kept me up all night. She is teething, and I feel bad for her."

"What did you do to help her?" I asked.

"I stayed up and rocked her and finally she went to sleep."

"Good!" I exclaimed. "You are a wonderful mother." The lady just beamed.

Many elderly people also love children and have a way of bonding with them. A young man who was barely educable would come each week to the elder care facility. He bonded with an elderly woman with dementia. It was so beautiful to see the two interact.

Aroma therapy:

- Take wash cloths and dip them into scented water, wring out well, microwave the cloth to warm it, and place on the resident's neck, hands, or face. Be sure the cloth is not too hot. Always ask the resident to feel the cloth before you put it around his/her neck.

Nature is close to the residents' hearts. Many residents I worked with had vegetable and flower gardens while living at home. Bring nature to them through fresh-cut flowers, leaves, tree branches, raspberries, strawberries, and fresh garden vegetables. Many used to can vegetables each season. I carried in all kinds of objects from nature. The hands-on (touch) and smells stimulate the residents. Many participated in the activity and enjoyed seeing, touching, and smelling the vegetables and flowers.

My mother grew beautiful, large roses while living in her home. She had taken great pride in nurturing her rose garden. She always lit up when she received a rose. She would smell it and reminisce about her rose garden. This made her feel good for the moment.

Therapeutic touch activity:

- Use soft, relaxing music in the background. Give the resident a hand massage, shoulder rub, and a foot massage after the person is relaxed enough to take the stimulation.

■ You can exercise and massage hands by filling a sock with sand and placing the patient's hand in the sock. Manipulate fingers in the sand. For a different sensation you can fill the sock with flour or leaves.

Sources of Stimulation

Environment: There is controlled and uncontrolled stimulation in the resident's environment. Their surroundings stimulate the basic senses and also their senses of emotions.

The patient can feel how you treat them through touch and tone of voice. People often try to make up for a lack of stimulation in the resident's environment. I have witnessed family caregivers that try to cover up for the Alzheimer's patient by finishing the patient's sentence or doing everything for the resident. They deny that the Alzheimer's patient has any problem at all.

This action on the part of the caregiver is picked up by the patient, and may prevent him/her from having the opportunity to maintain a daily sense of stimulation.

Also, stimulation comes from within the resident. The resident may not be able to speak but can feel pain and hear voices. Remember the hearing is the last to go in most human beings. Bear in mind that hearing, seeing, tasting, and moving all come under the umbrella of feeling. These are feelings that happen during the waking hours to make up sensory input. If the resident is restricted, he/she will lose contact with reality.

Work diligently to keep the Alzheimer's patient's life vital at their level and let them enjoy the moment.

Validation vs. Reality Orientation

Use the words *who, what, when, where,* and *how* to converse with an Alzheimer's patient, **but never *why*.** The patient has lost the ability to rationalize his or her actions. Asking *why* will only confuse the patient, and at any rate they should no longer be held accountable.

One day, when my mother was in the early stages of Alzheimer's, she asked me to feel the big lump on her head. I asked her how she'd gotten the lump, and she said she had hit her head on the cupboard door. "When did this happen?" I asked.

"I think yesterday," she replied.

"Is the lump really big?" I asked.

"Oh, yes," she said.

I asked her to show me where the lump was. She pointed to the middle of her head. I touched the spot and said, "Yes, that is a very big lump."

Actually, there was no lump. But it was important for me to validate her. She smiled; she knew there wasn't a lump. I told her that it would get better really soon, and I loved her even with a big lump on her head. She accepted this very nicely.

Reality orientation is correcting someone who is disoriented. It is fine to correct the patient about the time, where they are, and who their family and friends are, but it would have only irritated Mom if I had said, "No, you don't have a lump." She was grieving the loss of her memory. This is where validation versus reality orientation is most appropriate.

While working at a local care facility, I met a patient named Liddy. She was in the facility's kitchen one day, and she became combative. It became apparent that the caregiver with her was on her turf. Liddy ordered the caregiver out of her kitchen, and the caregiver tried to argue with Liddy, insisting that it wasn't Liddy's kitchen. Liddy only became more insistent and angry. I stepped in and told Liddy we'd get out of her way immediately. I talked the caregiver into leaving. I then said to Liddy, "You must be very tired. Were you working in your kitchen all day? Maybe you were expecting company."

"Yes," she said.

"Who came to visit?"

"My bridge club," she said. "It was my turn. I wanted everything to be perfect for my friends."

"What did you fix for them?" I asked.

"Chicken salad. I always use a fresh-cooked chicken," she replied.

I said, "You seem very tired. Let me get you a cup of coffee. Would you like to take a break? I would like to help you." She sat with me as we drank our coffee, then she let me help her clean up. My point is every staff member needs to be tuned in with the residents for their best interest and care. I was able to stop an upsetting confrontation by using validation. Every caregiver needs to learn validation techniques and should apply them in each appropriate situation.

I visited a care facility at Easter time. One patient thought it was Christmas. I asked the patient, "What is your favorite Christmas song?" She told me, and we sang it together.

"What does the song remind you of?" I asked.

"My husband," she replied. "He was very tall with coal-black hair. We sang this song every Christmas with our family."

Reality orientation only causes problems because in the patient's mind what he/she is thinking at the time is correct. Straightening out the Alzheimer's patient's thinking process will not work. Try to get into their world and walk hand-in-hand with the patient, linking them to wherever they are at for that moment, and at their level. How you approach the person and the situation can help keep the person happy, or cause chaos between the patient and the caregiver. Remember, the patient is living in the past. Their short-term memory is the first to go. The long-term memory stays intact for quite some time. Accept the changes in your loved one as the disease progresses.

In order to use the validation technique properly, you need to study validation and practice applying the techniques. It takes some work and some fast thinking but is worth it for your own sanity, and for the patient's mental well-being. Trust me, validation really works.

My mom washed dishes at her restaurant for many years. After she retired, she continued to wash dishes daily in her home. Since this was part of her routine, it was good to have her continue. However, as she moved into the second stage of Alzheimer's, she could no longer remember to put soap in her dishwater. So, rather than scolding her or confronting her, I would put the soap in the water in advance. She would then wash and rinse the dishes. I found it interesting that she could remember to rinse and dry the dishes, but couldn't remember the soap. She felt very useful and important because she knew she was helping.

She could also fold clothes, because this was also a routine task from her past. However, she didn't remember where the folded clothes went, so the family would help out by putting them away.

I can't tell you enough how important it is to be patient with your loved one with Alzheimer's and to work at their level. Prepare yourself to adjust your expectations as the disease progresses. Expect nothing and rejoice when the patient completes a simple task. Compliment them for their accomplishments. A caregiver needs to have knowledge and virtue to carry out their caregiving duties to the best of their abilities.

Helping to Jog the Memory

One day in March I brought a huge icicle to the care facility where I was working. I thought that the icicle would be great for feeling the cold temperature. I discovered more. All of the residents enjoyed seeing and touching the icicle. A resident said, "I remember on the farm how icicles formed all the way across the house. I was afraid to walk under those icicles for fear one might fall and hit me. That was before we had gutters to catch the water running off the rooftops."

One said, "I loved the glassy look on the icicles hanging down."

Another resident said, "I liked the various sizes of each icicle."

One of the men said when they were kids, they used the icicles for swords. This simple item became a wonderful tool to jog their memory.

Another time, I brought in a tape with the sound of the wind. One resident identified with the March winds. Another day I brought in some snow and made snowballs with them. They enjoyed the snow greatly. I asked the residents what they liked best about the snow. One woman said she enjoyed laying her whole body into the snow and flapping her arms up and down to make an outline of her body. She used her hands and arms to show how she did this as she exclaimed, "Oh say, how wonderful that was to be in the snow." She was smiling the whole time, and her eyes sparkled like diamonds.

I can recall picking my mother up one day from the group home when I had my catering business. She always talked about wanting to see a party that I catered. I asked permission from my client to let my mom see my setup. She arrived with me about one hour before the party to witness the setup. She held my hand as we walked around the area. She told my client, "You have a lovely home and lots of nice food." While my mom never remembered me taking her to the party it was a joy for me to see her smiling eyes. Memories of her 80th birthday party were brought back with that visit. I was thrilled.

One of the residents had a craving for shrimp, so I asked the nurse if I would be allowed to bring in six shrimp for her. With permission I arranged and delivered the shrimp. The resident was happy and enjoyed every bite. The taste helped her recall going out for shrimp with her husband.

One of the ladies wanted to help me bake. She could not remember how to crack an egg so, I said, "You can crack that egg. We will do it together." She was thrilled to have helped me crack the egg. She talked about how she gathered eggs on her farm.

Another resident wanted to run her sewing machine just to make a seam. She had been a wonderful seamstress in her time. Her daughter brought in her mother's sewing machine. I set it up and got it running. It was a joy to make her wish come true. This helped her remember the dress she had made for the ball she and her husband attended.

The Importance of Reminiscing

Reminiscing is fondly recalling memories, remembering for pure pleasure the happy experiences in life. Reminiscing is something that an Alzheimer's patient can do. Even though the short-term memory is destroyed by the disease, the long-term memory is still intact.

Reminiscing serves several functions. Life review reminiscence involves analyzing, evaluating, and coming to terms with unhappy life experiences, what is often termed "unfinished business," in someone's life. Naomi Feil does an excellent job with her videotape and book *The Validation Breakthrough* on using this technique to help people come to terms with unresolved issues.

When Vera was a little girl, she was repeatedly raped in the chicken coop by an older brother. She told no one, though the experience left her with an undying hatred of men all her life. It was only decades later when, as an Alzheimer's patient in a care facility, she became hysterical when a male nurse tried to help her. She screamed and struck out at the nurse. "Don't let him hurt me! He's going to attack me!" When he left the room, a female caregiver came to talk with her and ask what had happened. "He attacked me when I was a little girl!" she cried. As the caregiver continued to ask further questions, it became clear that Vera was describing her terrifying ordeal as a child. As she talked, Vera broke down and cried, finally able to release the pent-up emotions of a lifetime.

Annie, the oldest of eight children, had fallen in love with Herman, and they had made plans to be married. But times were hard in the Depression years, and the wedding kept being delayed as she worked to help support her family. Herman was called into the service and was killed in the line of duty. She grieved for him all her life, never marrying. At age 82, suffering from Alzheimer's, she called out for him. "Herman! Please come back to see me! You left me! How could you desert me? I need you!" The pain remained as fresh as it was decades ago.

One researcher wrote that he believes life review reminiscence is a part of healthy aging. Those suffering from depression can especially benefit from reminiscing; it helps the person adapt to the situation, come to terms with the past, and become more satisfied with life. I believe my mother distorted the past to help her remove some of the pain she endured in her life. It helped her get through her days.

As the elderly come to the close of their lives, reminiscing is a good way for them to reflect on their life experiences, to rethink what they have seen, done, and accomplished. It isn't always a sad process; it can also bring serenity, peace, and a sense of closure.

There are different forms that reminiscence can take:

■ Informative/recreational reminiscence: factual recall, perhaps using visuals to help the group reminisce about what they see.

■ Story-telling reminiscence.

■ Life review: a form of evaluative reminiscence.

■ Defensive reminiscence: a form which glorifies the past and indicates that there may be an unhealthy adjustment to the present.

A Reminiscence Group

I have several examples of positive reminiscence group activities on topics such as canning, making wishes, apples, school days, the farm, leaves, and the seasons of the year, in the second section of this book. Music is an effective way to jog memory and it has a calming effect as well.

A reminiscence group is a structured group activity in which the leader helps and guides the group members as they recall experiences, and leads them to affirm the value of the experiences. It can be done only as a conversation, but it is enhanced by adding props, playing songs, or using items with memory-evoking tastes, smells, or sounds. I am awed by the power of music to stimulate memories. Songs linked with important life happenings can unlock a kaleidoscope of associations, thoughts, and reflections. When you add music to an activity, the people who normally don't participate will light up and chime in with the discussion. It is wonderful to observe.

I have found that most residents gain great pleasure from recreational reminiscing and storytelling reminiscing. A rich and vivid reminiscence group experience with sensory detail makes the resident think the experience is immediate once again. Besides pleasure, reminiscence groups can create the following positive outcomes:

■ Improve self-esteem.

■ Boost life satisfaction.

■ Put the person in a positive frame of mind.

■ Encourage socializing in a positive climate.

Your tone of voice, enthusiasm, and approach all set the mood of the resident. Be sure you keep the resident feeling good about the group and set a non-threatening atmosphere. If the patients are in a social setting with a lot of stress or uncertainties, they can feel threatened and that can work against the purpose of the activity.

The setting:	Have the group meeting the same place each week, a comfortable, quiet area free from distractions. Make it look as home-like as possible. Set people in a half circle or around a round table (a round table is best for conversation). Use colorful fabrics or a centerpiece associated with the topic to get the discussion started. Make it feel, as much as possible, as if the people are just friends gathering over a cup of coffee.
Time:	30 to 60 minutes once or twice a week. I go to a facility once a week at the same time. The residents light up as I pull my accordion out of my box. "Oh, it is the accordion lady! We are going to have music!" Twice a week is better; the repetition is positive for Alzheimer's patients.
Group size:	Two to eight people is best, but it can work with up to 20 people sitting around tables or in a half-circle. The group I work with once a week has 8 to 12 people. I can manage that group fairly comfortably with one assistant.
Evaluating:	How well did the residents participate? Did they respond with interest?
Goals:	Maintain existing levels of functioning. Create happiness.

My Experience Leading Reminiscence Groups

You must constantly adjust as you go to meet the group's needs. I sometimes plan something that simply doesn't work out. One time I tried the topic of dreams. I got no response. But when I moved from dreams to wishes, the group came to life.

I have found that a prop such as an apple, greeting card, or flowers often piques their interest.

Introduce props one at a time; showing all of them at once can be overwhelming and increase difficulties with concentration and decision-making.

When I do a food-related topic, I play "My Favorite Things" from "The Sound of Music." I ask them, what is your favorite food? They usually mention sweets or ice cream. A fun song like "I scream, you scream, we all scream for ice cream," gets them smiling. Then we serve ice cream.

At the end, close the group with some social time. Serve coffee or juice. You can continue the conversation about the topic. Be sure to return the residents to the present moment—bring them back to reality. I always shake hands at the end of the activity and tell them to have a great day. As the group leader, you are responsible for helping them bridge from the group back to their daily routine. It's also important not to overstimulate the group. Overstimulation can disorient them.

The Importance of Preserving Dignity

Webster's Dictionary states, "dignity is worth, excellence…the quality of commanding esteem, to insist on being treated with respect."

Dignity is usually given to the frail or dependent elderly person by the caregiver, family, and friends. In addition, strangers should also enhance each elderly person's dignity. The caregiver cannot continue to think of independence as a strength but must focus on where the dependent person is in their time of life. Accent the positive for best results. Work with the person, making him/her feel good for the moment. Give that person a chance to feel joy and a sense of self-worth, telling the person he/she is important. Compliment them often for the little things they do or how they look. I found that just holding my mom's hand and telling her how lucky I was to have her with me made her feel good. I firmly believe that maintaining the resident's self esteem and self worth to bring the joy of the moment is very much a part of dignity. Let them do a task if possible, without rushing them. So what if it's not done perfectly? What matters is considering the patient's feelings and letting him/her know their life has value.

My mother's dignity was an important issue to me. I worked diligently with Mom's caregivers in the group home to make sure Mom was treated with respect. I let friends and neighbors know Mom had Alzheimer's. She wasn't herself any longer, and she did not always know what she was saying. I found it easy to extend my respect to Mom since I was educated about Alzheimer's. This enabled me to give my mom the dignity she so deserved. Her words and actions were a result of the disease. Because she was my mother I loved her no matter what. Hence, I used my head and heart to preserve her dignity. As the disease progressed, her memory was diminishing, and she was reverting back to childlike ways. However, I recognized she was an adult. I did not make her accountable because she no longer knew the difference and did not have reasoning power.

One time I took Mom to visit my husband's mother. My mom fed the birds. She said she was "feeding the chickens." We all complimented Mom for doing a good job of feeding the chickens. The chickens were so lucky to have a nice lady like Mom looking after them. She wore a big grin and I could tell she felt really good about this task. (I might add Mom had grown up with chickens.)

While I was playing my accordion at a care facility, a gentleman was in the audience who was very crippled and was in a geri chair. He had a tube in his throat to drain mucus. Some of the mucus came out of the tube. The caregiver attended to him immediately and cleaned him up. She covered the area and fussed over him. She held his hand and I could see his eyes brighten. She treated him with respect. That made me feel good. That caregiver let this man know he was all right. I had a real sense that this resident was treated with great respect.

On the other hand I witnessed a family member yelling at her mother because her mom would not follow her instructions. If a caregiver is frustrated and stressed out, she needs to take a deep breath and start over, keeping in mind the patient's dignity. Unfortunately the patient does not know any better and yelling does not help the resident, or the caregiver, in this case.

Dignity results from the kind interaction of the caregiver. It is just as hard for the patient to become dependent as it is for the caregiver to watch the person become dependent. Remember the dependent person is counting on your kindness and love.

Allowing the Alzheimer's patient to hold onto the past just may get the patient through the day, and the future days ahead. It helps the patient say I am okay. The past gives the patient perspective. They have no perspective of the present; their holding on to the past anchors them as a person. Patience, kindness, and interacting versus reacting to the Alzheimer's patient's words and actions will help keep the caregiver's sanity and in the long run preserve the Alzheimer's patient's dignity. I found myself doing a lot of laughing with Mom. Joking around helped Mom and me both get through our days. I remembered my mom's mind was very frail. She depended on me to be there for her.

If a caregiver has feelings of resentment and regrets the task of caring for the person, pre-serving dignity may be out of the picture. The caregiver must be sensitive to the person to meet their emotional and physical needs. With this generous act of kindness the elderly will be treated with dignity. Remember, the dependent elderly person has emotions until their dying day. Serve them with love and honor their dignity.

Alzheimer's Patients and Eating Disorders

Mom always liked chocolate chip cookies. Actually, she loved sweets in general, but her favorite cookie was chocolate chip. She generally made double batches of cookies. One afternoon while she was still residing in independent living we made a double batch of cookies. I put 24 cookies into her cookie jar and bagged up the rest to store in the freezer. In the evening after I thought she was tucked in bed and sleeping, I too fell asleep. I was exhausted and did not wake up until morning. I found an empty cookie jar and a dirty coffee pot. She had eaten all 24 cookies and had finished off a whole pot of coffee. She actually made the coffee and even pulled the plug. I was grateful for that. At first I thought that maybe she might have hidden the cookies in drawers, something Alzheimer's patients frequently do. I quietly searched drawers and cabinets. The cookies indeed were all gone. I asked, "Mom where are the cookies?" "What cookies?" she asked. I said, "The cookies we made yesterday." She said, "We never made any cookies yesterday." At that point I did not argue and realized that she had eaten all 24 cookies and did not remember her actions. It was a real learning experience for me to think that she couldn't remember making or eating the cookies. She did not get sick or suffer any real problems from her great binge. I did not bring up the topic to her again. However, I put only two or three cookies at a time in the cookie jar from then on. I was very curious about this episode. I talked to the nurse and social worker in our town. They assured me that was part of the disease. Some people with Alzheimer's never know when to stop eating and others refuse to eat.

Then I met another woman in the same complex. I told her my story. Her husband too had Alzheimer's. She said she set a one-pound box of unwrapped chocolate malted balls out in a big candy dish. Her husband ate six at a time. She moved the dish and he found them at night. He ate the whole pound. She too never put all the candy out at once after that. Unfortunately they can't remember what they ate and don't know when to stop eating.

By contrast, a lady in a care facility simply stopped eating. The caregivers could not get her mouth open to feed her; she had to go to the hospital where the staff fed her intravenously. My mother ended up the same way. She went from bingeing to not eating at all. I was able to feed her broth and liquids. She insisted she'd just eaten. It is heartbreaking to watch because you know the lack of nourishment means a slow death. My mother had been a very large lady with a hearty appetite. She used to love to go out to eat at buffets and enjoyed every morsel of food. She liked to cook and work in the kitchen. She spent many hours in her kitchen making bread and cookies. This dreadful disease stripped Mom of the privilege of enjoying the little things she loved, not to mention her memory. It also took away the emotional tie between a mother and daughter. I am not bitter, but sad for us both because she was such a part of my life. Fortunately, I have God in my life. I worked diligently on a daily basis to accept the things I cannot change, and to change the things I can, and I acquired the wisdom to know the difference. As I continued to laugh with her to stop my tears, I learned to understand she did not know the difference as the disease progressed and for her that lack of awareness was a gift. That thought lessened my emotional pain. As I reflect I now understand the real meaning of true love of a daughter and mother relationship. My love for her helped me to go on and help others.

Dementia and the Driving Dilemma—a Caregiver's Concern

With the increase of dementia, due to seniors living longer in the U.S., driving issues have become a big concern. Only a few states have laws restricting the driving by persons with dementia. Hopefully, that will change in the near future. Physicians in California are obligated to report cases of dementia. Missouri passed legislation to deal with drivers with dementia. The Alzheimer's Association in our area formed a committee to increase awareness in the community about this issue. A three-hour seminar was held in a local care facility, featuring a panel that addressed several issues of driving with dementia. The panel consisted of a nurse from the Department of Transportation, a neurology nurse, an occupational therapy (OT) driving specialist, an attorney from a personal injury law firm, an insurance agent, a police social worker and a Department of Aging and Transportation coordinator. I spoke at this seminar, representing family members dealing with Alzheimer's patients and driving issues. The Alzheimer's Association did an excellent job putting together a successful program.

Some of the information I absorbed from the panel was eye-opening. From a medical perspective, we were reminded that aging has several common effects on the human body: reflexes slow down, and some hearing and vision loss is common. Cognitive changes and chronic medical conditions can affect the elderly's driving skills. Alzheimer's disease has a great impact on cognition and physiologic change. The problem lies with who should be responsible to observe and report the driving behavior of the person with dementia. Often family members are reluctant because the burden may fall on them to shuttle the parent around. Family members may live out of town. Social workers can make suggestions but need the support of the family to convince the Alzheimer's patient not to drive and encourage them to find other means of transportation. Health care professionals are becoming more involved in raising the driving issue with families.

The Alzheimer's Association handed out a flyer (*Alzheimer's Disease/Caregiving Issues: Driving*) at the program. It states that in order to drive, a person must be alert, be able to make fast decisions, and react quickly. So a driver must be capable of being attentive and have sharp senses. Caregivers should watch over the person with dementia. Watch for warning signs of unsafe driving, such as not remembering how to find familiar places, not following traffic signals, making bad driving decisions, driving too fast or too slowly, becoming upset, and or confused while driving.

Driving is a privilege. There is a great stigma attached to the loss of driving privilege in the U.S. because driving represents independence and mobility. The person feels bad because he/she now needs to depend on family, friends, and other means of transportation to get around. The dementia patient often will hang on to the car keys because they do not want to ask for help.

Some approaches by caregivers to stop the person from driving may be as follows:

- Ask a doctor to write a "do not drive" prescription.
- Keep the car keys hidden.
- Disable the car by removing the distributor cap or battery.
- Park the car at a neighbor's home.
- Have the person tested by the Department of Motor Vehicles.
- Arrange for someone to drive your loved one where he or she wants to go.
- Substitute the person's driver's license with a photo identification card.

One of my friends told me that to stop his mom from driving he rigged up the horn on the car so it would blow obnoxiously loud until his mom turned off the keys. It scared her enough to stop her from driving. He only did this after trying to sensibly discuss her loss of driving skills with her. Reasoning power and examples did not work in his case.

The Alzheimer's Association suggests that it is very important to be sensitive and supportive when the person with dementia no longer drives. My mother became very angry and depressed when she was no longer permitted to drive.

A Test of Driving Skills

An AARP bulletin put out in the late 1990s suggests that a person should test one's driving skills. There are several warning signs:

- Have you had one or more minor accidents in the past two years?
- Do you have trouble making left-handed turns across traffic?
- Do you get lost easily? Can you follow directions easily to get to your destination?
- How are your reflexes?
- Have you run a red light or stop sign in the last two years?
- Have passengers told you that your driving makes them nervous?
- Do you take drugs, painkillers, sleeping pills, or antihistamines?
- Do you have problems with brief numbness, loss of function on one side of your body, or slurred speech?
- Do you have heart disease, diabetes, Parkinson's disease, epilepsy, or other medical problems?
- Do you have problems seeing while driving at night?

If you have answered yes to any of the above questions, it is wise to see your doctor.

It is probably good to mention that there are reversible causes of dementia such as reactions to certain types of drugs, emotional disorders, metabolic disorders, ear dysfunctions, nutritional deficiencies, tumor and trauma, infections, arteriosclerotic complications (i.e., myocardial infarction, stroke, or heart failure).

The above information was also handed out at the driving seminar. The Department of Transportation makes a decision about the person's driving ability on the individual signs, symptoms, behaviors, and the observations of others, not the type of condition or diagnosis. Confusion, disorientation, memory loss, impulsive behaviors, and poor judgment are very common signs of impairment. The Department of Transportation may require a road test, written test, medical report, and/or a vision exam or screening. They may take no further action or may order a cancellation of the license. The doctor makes the final judgment by signing a behavior report to support immediate cancellation of a license. Too often a police officer picking up an elderly person for a traffic violation sees his parent or a family friend behind the wheel and lets the person go. Workers in a driver's license testing division may feel sorry for the elderly person and slip the person through the process. The personal injury lawyer at the seminar made it clear that the impaired driver does get prosecuted for accidents and it can be very expensive and devastating. The lawyer handed out information that clearly states that the patient with dementia has the duty to drive carefully just like any other drivers on the road.

Caregivers' and Family Members' Exposure to Liability

There are state laws that forbid a person from authorizing or knowingly permitting an unlicensed person to drive a car under his control. The legal system owes a duty to the general public, and can take a broad view of responsibility to the ward, including relatives and others who have a special relationship to the patient, prosecuting them for allowing patient access to a car.

The "Deep Pocket" Rule

The insurance agent at the seminar I attended said, "The [insurance] company is like the wife—always the last to know." There isn't much the company can do to stop people from driving. There are no laws in effect that give insurance companies any authority to take away the car keys.

The occupational therapy driving specialist can give tests to the elderly to confirm driving skills. However, insurance does not cover these tests, and they can be very costly. Seniors are also sometimes reluctant to take this type of test because they fear losing their driving privileges.

My mother was very independent. I can still see her with her hands on the wheel with star-bright eyes and a glowing face. She carried her big black purse everywhere she went. She would pick up her friend for church and go out to eat afterwards for lunch. She loved to shop at her favorite grocery stores looking for the latest bargains. It was a way of life for her. Taking away the car keys was like a death sentence to her. Her emotions ran high when she could no longer drive.

I began to notice the change in Mom's driving skills a couple of years before she stopped driving. One April in the early to mid-1990s Mom decided to drive from her home in Indiana to Wisconsin to visit with us. April was far enough into spring that we should have not have had to worry about snow. The day she drove to Wisconsin we had a bad snowstorm that started late in the afternoon. I received a call from Mom: "Pat, come and get me right now." She quickly hung up the phone without telling me where she was.

I prayed for about 20 minutes and hoped she would call again. Finally the phone rang again. "Hi, this is your mother. Where are you? I told you to come and get me; I am in the ditch." I pleaded, "Mom, please don't hang up on me. Where are you?" She said, "I am at a lady's house." I finally got my mother to put the lady on the phone and I got the woman's phone number and directions to her house. I called my husband and we drove there and got

my mother's car out of the ditch. I got a tongue-lashing when I arrived for not coming sooner. At that point I did not try to reason with her. I just took her back to our home.

I was willing to drive her back to Indiana but she would not let me. She was very stub-
born and vehement about the whole situation. After a couple of days the roads were clear. I
took her out on the road and checked her driving ability. She seemed all right. I gave in and
she did make it home safely. I was relieved.

Six months went by, and Mom basically drove around her hometown. I continued to ask
local friends about her driving ability. As I have mentioned before, parents have a way of fool-
ing adult children when they fear losing their independence. I called long distance often and
Mom would make sense and sound okay. I had neighbors and my aunt check on her daily. I
did not get any bad reports from the neighbors on her driving ability at that point. My mother was not an easy person to deal with on the driving issue. She insisted she had her right to
drive and did not see driving as a privilege. I talked to her about my concerns about her driving ability.

For Thanksgiving she decided to drive to another sister's home. That was a 400-mile trip.
I was not happy that she was attempting that alone. I alerted my sister, and she thought Mom
would be fine. After all, Mom always drove alone to all of our homes. She got lost again and
my sister had to drive her home. I insisted that she could not drive any more long-distance
trips alone.

One year later the neighbor was riding with her as she ran a stoplight and two stop signs
on her normal routine errands. The neighbor also reported that Mom had gotten lost going to
the local grocery store. At that point the neighbor said that she refused to ride with her any
longer. I checked on her again and confronted her with the problem of running lights and getting lost. She denied that she'd done any such thing. I told her I loved her and feared for not
only her safety but also for the safety of other drivers and pedestrians. She became infuriat-
ed. I again backed off.

One day she was driving with another neighbor, and she hit a man on a motorcycle. No one was seriously injured, but I took the car away after that. Mom and our family could have been sued for everything. At that point I called the insurance company. They told me that Mom didn't have valid insurance nor a driver's license for the previous six months! She had not gone to the motor vehicle department to renew her license and she had let her car insurance lapse. At that point I had a doctor examine my mother and he confirmed she was in the early stages of Alzheimer's. I took the keys away and never let her drive again—against my mother's and the entire family's wishes. It had become a safety issue for all involved in this situation.

I brought her back to Wisconsin. She became very angry and nasty. She yelled at me and cursed me: "I am little Orphan Annie with no wheels! It is all your fault." At that point she called me "a mean son of a bitch." I swallowed hard and said, "Mom I love you with my whole heart and soul, and I will never let you drive again for your own safety and that of everyone else on the road. I will drive you anywhere your heart desires." She began to scream louder. I threw my arms around her as tears rolled down my cheeks. I kissed her cheek and said, "Well, little Orphan Annie, I would like to take you for ice cream but I guess I will have to return home and put you in a corner for being nasty." I pleaded and said, "Mom, please understand. You protected me and guided me when I was a little girl; now as your daughter I must protect you. It is a safety issue." She hung her head down for a couple seconds. It was the last time she ever gave me trouble about not being able to drive.

As a caregiver and daughter I had no choice but to take the keys away. I would have taken away the keys sooner if other family members hadn't protested so bitterly. Taking the keys away was one of the hardest chores to accomplish. A friend drove Mom's car away and sold it. We put the money into her account for her future health care. I plead with every caregiver not to wait for an accident to happen before taking away the car keys. You may not be so lucky as my family. You may be sued for negligence. It is your duty to take action when the parent is no longer capable of driving. In my case all the warning signs were there. I felt it was my responsibility to act. Too often a family member waits until there is an accident and then acts. Don't wait to take car keys away from a person who gets lost while driving, cannot read or follow road signs, or follow the speed limit. If you are riding with a person who needs directions to familiar places, please take action for every person's safety. A caring son or daughter will act in the name of love for the parent.

Survival Tip: Keep a Sense of Humor and a Good Attitude

"The longer I live, the more I realize the impact of attitude on life. Attitude, to me, is more important than facts. It is more important than the past, than education, than money, than circumstances, than failures, than successes, than what other people think, or say, or do. It is more important than appearance, giftedness, or skill. It will make or break a company…a church…a home. The remarkable thing is we have a choice every day regarding the attitude we will embrace for that day. We cannot change the fact that people will act in a certain way. We cannot change the inevitable. The only thing we can do is play on the one thing we have, and that is our attitude."

—*Charles Swindoll*

The Trouble Tree

The carpenter I hired to help me restore an old farmhouse had just finished a rough first day on the job. A flat tire made him lose an hour of work, his electric saw quit, and now his ancient pickup truck refused to start. While I drove him home, he sat in stony silence. On arriving, he invited me in to meet his family. As we walked toward the front door, he paused briefly at a small tree, touching the tips of the branches with both hands. When he opened the door he underwent an amazing transformation. His tanned face was wreathed in smiles and he hugged his two small children and gave his wife a kiss. Afterward he walked me to the car. We passed the tree and my curiosity got the better of me. I asked him about what I had seen him do earlier. "Oh, that's my trouble tree," he replied. "I know I can't help having trouble on the job, but one thing for sure, troubles don't belong in the house with my wife and the children. So I just hang them up on the tree every night when I come home. Then in the morning I pick them up again. Funny thing is," he smiled, "when I come out in the morning to pick 'em up, there ain't nearly as many problems as I remember hanging up the night before."

—*Author unknown*

Chapter 5:

Abuse and Fraud

Aging in America

In the beginning of the 1900s only 3.1 million Americans were 65 or older. That was only four percent of the population. In the United States by the early 1990s, 31.8 million people lived to a ripe old age. That is approximately one in every eight Americans. The over-65 population is projected to soar to 65 million by 2030. In 1910 life expectancy was 53.

Women outlive men by a ratio of 154:100. If you visit nursing homes you will realize in a hurry that most of the residents are female. About 56 percent of elderly men and 36 percent of elderly women live with their spouses; 12 percent of the elderly live with their children or a family member. About one third of elderly men and women live alone.

In the early 1990s the median income of older persons was about $14,000 for men and $8,189 for women. The median income for the over-65 population was about $10,000. In the 75-plus age group, approximately one in ten men and one in five women live in poverty. That's hard to believe in such a rich country as America.

Caring takes energy. But in our society, old people often are considered useless. Many people wonder when the old folks are finally going to die—after all, the elderly have nothing to contribute to society any longer. That is where the family must pitch in and keep the elderly person feeling wanted, loved, useful, and needed. Make the elderly person a part of the family and community as long as possible.

Abuse

Every person wants to be wanted, needed, and loved. Aged folks with late-stage Alzheimer's have the same needs as babies, but they are not cute like babies. Elder abuse is very serious because when an angry, unstable, or stressed-out relative or uncaring employee is in charge of that helpless senior, that elderly person may suffer abuse to the degree the care-taker wants him or her to. They are at the caregiver's mercy. Changing diapers, cleaning bottoms, and wiping up drool is expected when caring for a baby, but is not accepted by many adult children when caring for an aged parent and the disrespect shows. It is a must for every human being to use their energy to care for and about the elderly.

One of the greatest problems the elderly face is that abuse or neglect frequently goes unreported. This is especially true of abuse that occurs in a caregiver's home, for the elderly person may fear that he/she has no other place to go. A victim may be put in protective placement, but it is a long, drawn-out affair, especially if the court gets involved in the case. Protective placement services are provided by an individual or agencies for persons who can no longer manage their affairs, carry out normal activities of daily living, or protect themselves from abuse, neglect, or exploitation that may result in harm to themselves or others.

There is a toll-free hotline to report elder abuse: (800) 677-1116. Unfortunately when people report abuse it is not always thoroughly investigated. Many times, folks do not want to get involved in an abuse case. If you are concerned about the well-being of an elderly person and want to get involved, it is wise to know the difference between abuse and neglect.

Abuse is the infliction of physical, sexual, emotional, or financial injury or harm.

Neglect is:
◼ Failure to provide services when such failure presents either an imminent danger to the person's health, safety or welfare, or substantial probability that death or serious physical harm will result.
◼ Misappropriation of funds or property of in-home clients or residents in long-term care facilities.
◼ Falsified documents which verifies service delivery to in-home clients.

The above signs should be reported to your local aging department. You can give names of witnesses, but if the victim denies it or does not cooperate you are back to square one. Unfortunately, it just is not an easy task to report the abuse and have something done about it.

Usually a Division of Aging worker will investigate reports of the alleged abuse and neglect. Generally they will interview the reported victim, the witnesses, and the alleged perpetrator.

For example, a friend of mine knew her neighbor was being abused, so she reported it. The elderly person had Alzheimer's and was living with her son. The son was denying her care, falsifying records, and stealing her money. The son had threatened his mother that if she reported anything when the social worker came in, he would put her into a nursing home. So the mother was quiet.

Unfortunately when a social worker is called in, he or she may make an appointment weeks in advance and will have a staged visit, giving the abuser time to prepare. That defeats the entire purpose. Many aging departments are understaffed, underfunded, and overwhelmed with cases. Often social workers working in an aging department have their hands tied and can't help even if they want to.

It is hard for the social worker to keep up and do the best job under these kinds of conditions. It is easier to detect physical abuse and neglect than emotional abuse and neglect. The court systems throughout the United States aren't well equipped to deal with emotional abuse.

Review the five categories caseworkers will investigate for signs of abuse and neglect (taken from Missouri's Response System):

1. Physical appearance.
2. Client's environment.
3. Behavior of family or caregiver.
4. Social indicators.
5. Client's behavior.

There are many laws to protect the person who reports abuse or neglect. Doctors and nurses are also supposed to report abuse but often gloss over it for their own protection. At any rate, elder abuse is a crime and there isn't much being done by families, friends, or professionals to change this scene. The laws are in place, but they must be carried out in order to prevent elder abuse. It goes back to the people.

In the Fort Wayne, Indiana, area some residents have formed a group to help fight elder abuse. For example, there was the case of a diabetic mother who stayed with her son. He ignored her while collecting her Social Security check, supposedly to care for her. Since she was placed in a locked room she did not get the care she needed. When it was too late he took her to the hospital, but his mother died. The medical team reported him and he was prosecuted. With more watchdogs and efforts made by the medical staff in hospitals and nursing homes and neighbors and friends working together, there would be less abuse. Stiffer penalties and fines are needed. We can no longer take the approach, "Oh well, it is a family affair." We all need to be willing to get involved. We also need to teach our children to respect and help the elderly. If the law is not enforced and we don't work together on this horrible problem, it will only get worse. Since we work hard to help the elderly live longer we need to understand our duty to be kind to them. The body and mind of an elderly person may wear out, but they can still experience the emotions of sadness and happiness.

Elder Abuse Resulting From Parents Mixing Up Love With Money

The tendency to confuse financial support and love is a common pitfall for parents. They believe that they are being good parents by giving money to, and constantly helping out, their adult children. Without realizing it they take abuse from their adult children in the name of love. Adult children get into trouble and continue to expect their parents to bail them out. Often the adult child will insist that it is the parents' responsibility to help them and abuse the parents if they refuse the adult child's demands.

Too many parents who would never take that kind of abuse from a friend, neighbor, or stranger are willing to take it from sons or daughters. Parents are willing to excuse their adult children of their poor behavior and conduct. For example, a woman repeatedly asked to borrow money from her mother. Every time she borrowed money she promised that she would pay her mother back. She never did. Whenever the woman did not get her way she threw a temper tantrum. This technique worked every time.

Another parent would babysit for her son's children at a moment's notice—even when she had just returned home from the hospital with doctor's orders of bed rest. Some parents give up their plans to meet their children's demands without any notice. It is obvious that these adult children are very selfish and self-centered. Parents need to understand that money does not buy love.

When an adult child becomes used to using parents as a bank, they expect that service to continue forever, and when the parent grows older the adult child does not see a need to spend their parents' money on them for their health care. Instead, they may move their mom or dad into their own home, looking for every opportunity to "get their inheritance early." They may give very poor care to the Alzheimer's patient because the parent is clueless as to what is going on. This sad scenario can happen anywhere. Why? Parents living alone fear losing contact with their adult child. They feel giving in to them will keep the adult child coming back. Unfortunately the adult child comes back for all the wrong reasons, and parents lose out in the end.

Because my parents grew up in the Depression days, they were taught to forego the extra nice things. Mom was the only person working in her family and she supported every family member, paying the rent and putting food on the table. She waited two extra years to marry my father because she felt obligated to her family. This was not an uncommon practice back in the days of the Depression.

In today's society many adult children have two incomes, yet they often live beyond their means. When they need money, they go running to their parents. People who do this have no restraints or scruples about draining their parents' funds. They are not compassionate people but very self-serving. This type of person makes a poor caregiver. The parent has backed himself or herself into a terrible situation because they enabled that adult child to become very self-centered by supporting the needy, greedy ways of the adult child. It is very clear that money does not buy respect or love.

It has been my observation that fathers often practice tougher love with their adult children than mothers do. Fathers also fear being alone when they become elderly and feeble. The difference between a mother's and a father's fear is that Dad does not want to lose his wife. Fathers value their wives' companionship especially in their old age. Mothers frequently can't say no to the adult child's demands and thus they open themselves up for abuse.

Parents who do not set boundaries early in life often are the seniors that will not get good care from their children and will become abused.

Say no, emphatically, to the adult child that continues to insist on draining your finances for your future. There is an old saying, "demand respect and you will receive respect." Adult children need to understand that a family takes care of parents without any strings attached. Remember, the responsible adult child is the one who will make sacrifices in the best interest of his/her parents' care. It is the parents that set the tone for their care in their old age in many cases. Parents need to think hard about the potential problems of buying love and act accordingly to set the tone for their future of the so-called "golden years." The parents' actions toward their adult children in the early years may well seal their fate later in life.

Social Security

The Social Security Administration (SSA) has a 24-hour toll-free hotline: (800) 772-1213. If you have access to a computer, you can also visit their website at www.ssa.gov. The SSA treats all calls confidentially. For people who are hard of hearing or deaf, the Social Security

Administration has a toll-free TTY number, (800) 325-0778, which is answered between 7 a.m. and 7 p.m. on business days.

Keep in mind that the Social Security lines are busiest on Mondays and early in the month. You may get a busy signal or have to wait on the line for help. For better service call at other times. The Social Security office in your area can give you information about Medicare and Medicaid as well. Medicaid is for those on fixed incomes in need of financial help for medical services.

For the most part, the employees in the Social Security offices I have visited have been courteous and helpful. There are forms available to help a person do the job right. It is the representative payee (the person legally designated to handle the patient's Social Security funds) who must be honest and follow through for the sake of the beneficiary. The SSA is aware of the problem of fraud and is working to crack down on it.

For general information about Social Security and SSI (Supplemental Security Income) benefits, ask for a copy of the booklet *Understanding The Benefits* (Publication No. 05-10024).

The number for the SSA Fraud Hotline, used to report misuse or inappropriate use of funds, is (800) 269-0271. The address is SSA Fraud Hotline, P.O. Box 17768, Baltimore, MD 21235. If you have concerns (and written proof) that a representative is misusing a payee's Social Security check, call this number and ask for the Inspector General.

I recommend reading a booklet that you can obtain from your local Social Security office. It is called *Social Security: A Guide for Representative Payees*. It is SSA Publication No. 05-10076.

There is a form (OMB No. 0960-0014) that the representative payee must complete. The form asks, how will you, the representative, know the claimant's needs or does the claimant have a court-appointed legal guardian? What is your relationship to the claimant? Have you ever been convicted of a felony? (If yes, tell the truth.) The payee also has to tell their name, date of birth, and social security number. The Social Security Administration does try to get information to try to select the right representative payee.

Generally if the elderly person is competent, he or she and the potential representative can come in person to the Social Security office and fill out an application. If the doctor rules the elderly person incompetent due to a mental disease such as Alzheimer's, their designated power of attorney, or guardian of the person or estate, can become the representative payee. The SSA also expects the representative payee to fill out an annual report on how he or she has spent the funds on the ward. The representative payee must make sure that the elderly person's needs for food, clothing, shelter, and recreation are met. In addition, benefits can be used to pay for medical needs such as eyeglasses, hearing aids, and dentures not covered by Medicare, Medicaid, or private insurance. If a beneficiary is in a care facility, the representative payee should use the benefits to pay unusual charges for care. The Social Security office encourages the representative payee to set aside a minimum of $30 each month to be used for the beneficiary's personal needs or saved on his/her behalf. This can be placed in a checking or savings account called a "collective account." This $30 per person per month must be used for the beneficiary's personal needs.

If money is left over after meeting basic needs, it then can be spent on things that would improve the beneficiary's daily living conditions or provide better medical care. For example, you could use the funds for major health-related expenses such as a motorized wheelchair or supplemental insurance premiums. Perhaps an elderly person may get some pleasure from a magazine subscription or a movie or cable or a play. If you are not sure of special purchases ask the Social Security Office about such spending before you fulfill such obligations. For example, spending funds on expensive jewelry could make the beneficiary ineligible for payments.

Form SSA-623-F6, *Social Security Administration Representative Payee Report* is sent out to the representative payee to account for the spending. Unfortunately it is very general and does not require canceled checks or a great deal of details. This makes it very easy for family members to steal the funds from their parents who are incompetent, or competent and overly trusting.

While I have worked in the care facilities in Wisconsin and have traveled to other states for book signings, I have heard and witnessed horror stories about the representative payee stealing the elderly patient's monthly Social Security check. The problem lies in several areas. First of all, the parent does not want to report the adult child for fear of losing a place to stay or of not seeing that adult child again. The financial abuse just is not reported enough when it occurs.

The Social Security Administration does not have enough staff to spot-check for abuse. (I firmly believe if the representative payee had to return canceled checks and was required to keep a daily log of spending and finances it would help cut down the abuse.) There should be more investigators to follow up on reports of misuse of funds in a timely fashion. In my opinion, if the representative payee is suspected of stealing, then he or she should be required to come in within three days with proof of how funds are being spent. If you are doing your job as representative payee, you will have no problem showing this documentation.

A friend who lives and works in the South as a home health care person reported that the woman she cared for was abused. Her son came only once a month to see his mom, long enough to come and cash her Social Security check, and did not return until next month. The woman lived on practically nothing. No one could get her to speak up. While the home health person spoke up her hands were tied because there was a lack of cooperation from the beneficiary. The person advocating for the elderly is often asked to leave well enough alone.

Even if the Social Security Office believes funds are being misused, it takes months and even years for an investigation. Sometimes the Social Security office has to go back to the archives to get information on the representative payee report because that representative payee did not keep good records.

If you are a representative payee you must keep very good records. There are cases where family members are angry about the situation and may just report the representative payee out of spite. It is often hard for the person at the Social Security office to sort out the truth. Also, the Social Security office does not have a big staff to investigate all the cases. In some states investigators have been added to staff because this is becoming a problem for the Social Security office. In my opinion, background checks should be done on a representative payee when the beneficiary is incompetent. Having a direct-deposit account with your bank helps, too, as the money goes straight into your account and there's no need for a third party.

A Social Security check goes out once a month. The check is usually one month behind. For example, the check received in March is the payment for February. If the beneficiary dies, the representative payee must refund the check to SSA—even if the beneficiary dies on the last day of the month.

You must pay income taxes on Social Security benefits. In January of each year the Social Security Administration mails a Social Security Benefit Statement (Form SSA-1099) that shows the amount of benefits paid during the previous year. A tax accountant or family member in charge of taxes needs to prepare the statement and send the state and federal returns whether the beneficiary needs to pay or not. The government wants these checks accounted for each year. Keep in mind that as the representative payee, you must report changes such as if the beneficiary dies or moves, the beneficiary no longer needs a payee, or you are no longer responsible for the beneficiary. As payee, you are liable for repayment of money you receive on behalf of the beneficiary. If you do not report them and you are caught, you are in trouble!

One of the crimes that frequently occurs is the continued spending of the Social Security check after the death of the beneficiary. The representative payee must report the death to the Social Security Administration and must not cash checks on behalf of the deceased person. If you do so and are caught, you can be prosecuted. (And rightfully so—it is not your money.) When the beneficiary dies, the funds belong to the person's estate. A legal representative of the estate will handle the funds according to state law.

If you stop serving as the payee for a person receiving Social Security, you must notify the Social Security Administration immediately. You must return any benefits, including interest and cash on hand, to the SSA. These funds will be reissued to the beneficiary or to a new payee directly. Sometimes the SSA will ask that the funds be turned over to the beneficiary or to the newly designated payee.

For information on Medicare and Medicaid, call your local Social Security Administration office and ask for a copy of the *Medicare Handbook* (HCFA Publication 10050). It is important for the representative payee to keep correct and organized medical records.

Allegiance

The dictionary states that allegiance means loyalty owed by a citizen to a government, or loyalty to a person or cause.

What does the term allegiance have to do with the elderly's care? The answer is simple: Everything! Lucky is the elderly person that has a daughter, son, relatives, friends, caregiver, social worker, doctor, nurse, lawyer, or judge with a true sense of loyalty to them involved in their lives.

When a worker in the elder care field has a strong sense of allegiance he or she will do what is in the person's best interest. Unfortunately there are far too many cases where the elderly suffer because of too much money or lack of money. I will give you several examples.

While traveling around the United States I have spoken with several social workers. One social worker said that she can "only suggest." If the family members do not take her suggestions, her hands are tied; she is not allowed to enforce her ideas. Another social worker said, "The elderly have the right to choose which family member they want to live with." Even if the elderly person has Alzheimer's? She said, "Yes." A social worker cannot stop a caregiver who is abusing a patient; they can only report the abuser, and often the courts are too slow to act upon evidence of abuse.

One social worker reported that she had to go to a home for a visit. The elderly man's daughter was the guardian. The daughter sat in the living room holding her father's hand and pretending she was the loving daughter; in reality she was emotionally abusing her father behind closed doors. The daughter let her father die. The autopsy showed neglect. The daughter admitted after her father died that she was saving the inheritance for herself. Even worse, the daughter believed she was entitled to the funds and thought she was in the right for her immoral act. Her father did not know what was going on.

Judges more often than not rely on lawyers to tell them the story. There are many good and helpful lawyers, but there are some driven only by self-interest. If a lawyer who acts as an advocate only wants to make a lot of money off the elderly, he will persuade the judge to make a decision in his favor—not in the name of helping the elderly but because his allegiance is to his purse strings. Even worse, some judges do not even read the cases. Often there are thousands of cases, especially in a large city, and not enough judges or hours in the day to read every case. The average citizen doesn't realize this.

I talked to a lawyer at length and asked how he would feel if it were his mother being abused. He replied, "I would not abuse my mother. And when I try a case, it is just another case. I am totally emotionally detached. Now that you mention it, I guess I would become emotionally upset if someone was abusing my mother, and I had my hands tied so I could not help her. I never thought much about your questions before."

There are many good doctors that genuinely care about their patients. But with malpractice lawsuits, doctors too often are afraid to make the proper decision to help the elderly. Make sure you have a caring, concerned doctor helping you and your loved one.

Recommendations

■ Each person should prepare for old age early in life by getting their affairs in order and know whom to trust to care for them. Make wishes known in writing and choose a guardian who will follow through.

■ Clamp down on family members who abuse their parents and loved ones. Make accountability an issue.

■ Anyone applying for guardianship should be scrutinized with credit checks and background checks.

■ Abuse can come in many forms other than physical. Emotional abuse is easier to hide. Any suspected abuse needs to be investigated and not by scheduling home visits weeks in advance, giving suspected abusers time to clean up their act. Often, the abusing caretaker threatens to put the ward in a nursing home and abandon them. The ward takes the abuse out of fear.

■ Every community across the country needs a strong interfaith organization to help the elderly. We all need to band together to see that our seniors are getting proper care to help them live and die with dignity. We will all be there someday.

■ What I want to do most is to bring the focus of the public on these issues. This can be done through the media, with support from the court systems, and legislators—just to mention a few avenues. By sharing my experiences I have made a difference in my own community. It is awareness, education, and dialogue that will bring the changes.

■ Tap into resources already in the community. There are many good people out there wanting to help.

Elder abuse is a crime that cannot continue. Statistically, many of us will be elderly one day. Do you think such abuse can never happen to you? If so, think again.

There are elderly folks who have the financial resources to pay for good care, but still need a loving person to watch over them.

There are advocacy groups and lobbyists for the elderly who are doing good work. Though there are some safety nets in place within the judicial system to help prevent abuse, there is still not enough protection for our vulnerable elderly population.

Chapter 6:

Selecting a Care Facility

There are many wonderful adult children who are very interested in making the right decisions for their parent with Alzheimer's disease. Those decisions will probably change as the disease progresses. There are various levels of care available, and with a little research, you will be able to find one that suits the needs of your loved one.

Adult Day Care Centers

When the Alzheimer's patient is first diagnosed with early-stage dementia, one solution for a caregiver is an adult day care program, where a person can spend the day one to five times per week. This gives them an opportunity to socialize with other people their age and continue to be part of the community. There are many wonderful day care centers that have programs and activities to meet the early-stage patient's physical and emotional needs; some provide extra services, such as washing and setting hair. Those warm and fuzzy feelings are very important to the person's emotional well-being.

An adult day care center is a good way to start getting a person comfortable in a care facility setting. The elderly person must be considered before making any decisions. Some elderly people refuse to go to the day care center. You may have to stay with them at the center the first couple of times. It is an adjustment. Once they get started, they usually enjoy the activities and atmosphere and find they like being with other seniors. They enjoy the attention. It takes time to adjust to their new surroundings. People with Alzheimer's can become very confused in a new situation. Some may be frightened of this experience at first. If the family and the day care staff work together they can be instrumental in the adjustment period for the Alzheimer's patient.

John did not want to go to a day care center, and he told his daughter that the activity assistant was mean to him. After checking out the situation, she found that it was just the opposite. John was mean-spirited to the activity person. With hard work they got John to come around. Sometimes it takes time, love, and patience to accomplish the goals.

Often an adult day care center will not take your loved one if he or she is sexually aggressive or combative. They may not have a trained staff person to work with these types of behavior problems. Your loved one may be better cared for in an Alzheimer's unit or by trained staff who come to your home.

What to Look for in an Adult Day Care Center

- The facility is clean, attractive, and free of unpleasant odors.
- The building is wheelchair accessible.
- There is comfortable and sturdy furniture.
- There is a quiet place for conferences.
- Activities are offered throughout the day.
- There is extra volunteer help.
- A friendly and happy staff intermingles with the adults.
- Lunch should be provided if your loved one stays the entire day.
- Juice, water, coffee, snacks, and food for special diets are provided.
- Unexpected visits by family members should be welcomed.

When You Visit a Day Care Center, Keep These Things in Mind.

- Make an appointment and stay at least an hour to observe.
- Get references.
- If permitted, bring your loved one along on a visit to help them get started.
- Make sure you feel welcome.
- The environment should feel safe and non-threatening.
- There should be assistance for eating, walking, toileting, taking medications.

- Are there personal care services such as shampoos, bathing, and shaving?
- There should be mental stimulation.
- Ask questions about the center. (How long has it been in operation? Days open? Hours? Is there transportation to and from the day care center? Do they accept people with memory loss, incontinence, or limited mobility? Inspect the staff's credentials—how many staff work with how many seniors?)
- When you call the day care center ask for a brochure and an activity calendar.
- Be sure you are comfortable talking to the staff. If your loved one has memory loss, the staff can fill you in on the day. Sometimes you may ask your loved one what did you do today and the answer is, "Oh! nothing," or "I don't remember."

For information on The National Council on the Aging, Inc., call (202) 479-1200 or write NCOA/NIAD, 409 Third Street SW, Washington, D.C. 20004.

To find an adult day care center in your area call the Area Agency on Aging (AAA) at (202) 296-8130 to locate the AAA in your area. Also use your local Yellow Pages® to search for adult day care centers or aging services.

There are many difficult decisions to make when in charge of your loved one. One of the most difficult decisions for most adult children is to place Mom or Dad in a nursing facility. Some children promise their parents they will never be placed in a nursing home. But that may be a promise an adult child cannot keep because he or she cannot give proper round-the-clock care to an Alzheimer's patient. The adult child may have children of their own to care for or may not live in the area. To select the right care facility, start out by asking some simple questions.

- Does my loved one have trouble communicating?
- Does he/she need assistance going to the bathroom, getting dressed, or bathing?
- Does he/she need cues to perform certain tasks?
- Does he/she have unique behaviors such as wandering, combativeness, confusion, sexual aggressiveness, or withdrawal?

- Does he/she need someone to give him/her medication?
- Will he/she do better to have a private room or a shared room?
- What type of social activities would you want the care facility to offer?
- Do you want all three meals and snacks to be offered daily? And does your loved one have special dietary needs?
- Can you come and visit any time of the day without warning to the facility?
- Is it important to you to have your loved one placed in a setting that only cares for persons with dementia?
- How many caregivers are staffed for the number of people in that home?
- What are the costs of care in that facility?

Think it through very carefully and be honest to yourself and family about the amount of care required and the atmosphere desired for your loved one. Often a family caregiver fails to see the problems and will reason that the loved one is "not all that bad." Doctors can recommend tests that may help you decide which care setting is best.

Independent Living Facilities

Almost every community has facilities with different levels of care. There are complexes that provide independent living. These are apartments where most people with mild or no dementia can function fairly well. Independent living facilities require the resident to sign up for a certain number of meals per month. They often have bus service to the grocery store and offer many activities. When I travel and play music in an independent living arrangement most people seem fairly content. They make friends with other folks in the facility. They chat and play cards. Some folks share their talents by playing the piano and singing. Many have hobbies and belong to clubs. They volunteer in the facility's store or help arrange parties and do art projects. Most of them stay very active. This type of housing does not have to be licensed. A staff member does not have to be on duty 24 hours a day. This type of setting is also referred to as senior living, retirement housing, or senior apartments.

A friend who lived in a nearby assisted-living complex with round-the-clock staffing had a heart attack. She pulled the chain by her bed, and the rescue squad was there immediately. They saved her life. They told her if she had been living in her own home she would have died. When shopping for an independent living arrangement, you might want to consider a complex that offers regular apartments as well as units in an assisted living setting. When the person needs more care he/she can move to the next unit on the same campus. The patient can still have his/her own apartment or private room with more assistance to meet daily needs.

Assisted Living or a Group Home Setting

While shopping for a group home I had a list of needs and preferences for my mother. It was important that caregivers had training in dementia. I took notes on each care facility I visited. I made sure that the facility had the ability to meet my mother's needs before making any decisions. The facility I selected provided many services. They did her laundry and provided sheets and towels for her. They also required her to use their pharmacy choice. I had the time, so I did her hair because it was a good way to spend time with her.

When I moved my mom to a group home I made out a care plan for her and listed what type of assistance she would need from the caregivers. I also listed in writing her favorite foods. Each week I supplied extra ice cream for her so she could have that anytime she pleased (my mother had no diet restrictions). I had to work with her to get her to eat meals, and ice cream was my bargaining tool. Many assisted living facilities will let you bring in extra treats for your loved one. You also can bring in pictures and a few decorations to make them feel more at home.

24-Hour Care With Skilled Nursing Services

Nursing homes often like to be called health and rehabilitation centers or health care facilities, since the term "nursing home" has such frightening connotations for many people, especially the elderly. There have been many improvements since the old days. A good health care facility has 24-hour care and registered nurses on staff. A registered dietitian organizes the meals. Some residents need pureed foods due to swallowing problems. Other just can no longer chew their food properly. Swallowing can be a problem and there is a fear of aspiration. Aspiration occurs when food isn't swallowed and is instead sucked into the air passages where it blocks the airway.

There are structured activity programs for the residents. These activities keep the residents vital and stimulate them to keep them mentally alert. The skilled nursing homes are licensed by the state and federal government and must follow specific regulations.

A Doctor's Role

A doctor often visits a nursing home to examine patients. Whether a patient is living with family or in a care facility it is very important to keep constant communication open with your loved one's doctor. You need to stay on top of the overall wellness of your loved one. Most physicians encourage families to make sure that the loved one is getting physical exercise, eating properly, and taking their medicines. The doctor will advise that medications be monitored. The Alzheimer's patient generally does not remember taking the medicine and could overdose. That is one of the advantages of skilled nursing. The nurses on duty hand out the medications and chart it.

One patient loved to eat grapefruit for breakfast. But the directions on the patient's medication read, "Do not eat grapefruit with this medication. Grapefruit has a component that speeds up the pace of the medication in the bloodstream." Caregivers had to monitor the patient to be sure he was never given grapefruit, for his own protection. Family and staff must be aware of situations like this, and it must be included on the patient's chart.

The Importance of Visitors

I can't stress enough that once your loved one is placed in a facility (whatever level), please visit them. I can't believe how many adult children place their parents in a facility and never visit! The residents need so little to make them happy. That is one reason I find it such a joy to play my music and visit with the elderly. I once went to a facility's dining room and played dinner music as a strolling accordionist. As I walked around I spotted a gentleman tapping along with the music. I gave him a big smile. He broke down into tears. I bent down spontaneously and kissed him on the cheek and squeezed his hand. He said, "Thank you." I later learned no one visits him. It must be very tough to experience such loneliness and feelings of being forgotten.

As a family member I wanted to be confident that my mother was receiving the best care when I was not there. I watched how the workers handled mood swings and how medication was identified and monitored. I also came at a meal time and saw that the food was appetizing. I talked to a couple of residents too. I got a written list on the kind of assistance that was provided and also the cost. Activities are a must for Alzheimer's patients. They need to have that extra pleasure during their day to help them trigger memories of familiar activities from the past.

Many adult children go to the care facility and don't know what to say to their parent. As I mentioned before, just holding their hand and saying nothing is acceptable. Nursing homes that have the title "rehabilitation center" also offer respite care. If you are caring for a loved one in your home and need a break, make arrangements in advance to have your loved one stay a short term, such as a week, while you go on vacation. If your loved one is being released from the hospital and is not strong enough to go home, he/she can be sent to the rehab center and cared for until he/she is stronger.

Looking for an Alzheimer's Unit

If you are looking strictly for an Alzheimer's unit, ask to see their mission statement. Watch how the residents are being treated. Check out the cleanliness of the facility and the residents. Make sure you can stay involved in problem solving. Find out the type of care provided by the facility when the Alzheimer's patient is in late stages of the disease. Will the patient have to be moved as the result of the progression of the disease? In addition when visiting the facility look for books, posters, or brochures on Alzheimer's facilities. Try to find a recent report on Alzheimer's facilities and see how your choice rates. Look for a list of residents' rights and be sure the staff's allegiance is to protect those rights. Watch staff-resident interaction noticing how the staff treats residents. Observe to see if families can ask the staff questions. Check to see if the staff is asking the residents questions pertinent to each resident's interest.

Find out how many activities are offered each day and where the activities take place. I also came in when the activity director was working with the residents. Check to see if the residents are sitting around the nurses station or sitting in their rooms. One of the facilities I visited played Lawrence Welk over and over while I was there. Many residents were sleeping with the TV on. There is no stimulation in that situation. Find out the staff's qualifications. If the staff seems stressed out, beware. Is the staff friendly to you and the residents? Find out how many staff members there are, and at what times they're on duty. Check to see that the doors are secure, safety features are installed in the bathrooms and hallways, and lighting is adequate. Check for safe places for the person to wander both indoors or outdoors. Check for unpleasant odors. Make sure there are no unusual noises that will agitate the resident. Before you make a final decision about placement re-visit the facilities that are best suited for your loved one. I went back unannounced and my decision was a good one.

My best advice is to encourage family members to stay involved and continue to attend support groups. Share with families and friends and have your own little support group. Take care of yourself and do things you like to do too. If you don't take care of yourself, you won't be in any shape to take care of others. Learn to relax. Visit your loved one regularly and participate in activities. Participate in the care plan meetings and monitor what is going with your loved one.

Evaluating a Facility: Mission Statement vs. Reality

Each facility has a mission statement. While traveling around to various nursing facilities, I read many mission statements. Sometimes they are very lengthy, and I wonder if the staff is really following the promises of the mission statement. It's worth asking for a copy of their mission statement when you visit a care facility. Usually it is included on a brochure available from the marketing department.

A sample mission statement: "After 95 years of service, our mission is to continue to care for the elderly from the heart, responding to their needs in a holistic approach. Our care facility will treat each resident as an individual with dignity and serve them with love. Our care facility will continue to help make the resident feel comfortable in our home-like setting while providing services to meet the needs of each resident. Our care facility is committed to maintain their independence as long as possible, giving quality care and considering their emotional needs with respect."

You can't judge a book by its cover. Investigate to find out what the facility offers—the kind of environment, and the type of care that your loved one needs.

It is really people who make the difference. I provided music programs on several occasions at a private care facility. It was quite small and owned by the same people for 35 years. The facility was old and very simply decorated. The rooms were not fancy but they were cozy. There was plenty of help. Each time I went back, the same staff members were there. The residents were happy and smiling. I always enjoyed playing music at that facility. The residents had plenty to eat and were allowed to snack when they wanted to. They did little housekeeping chores with guidance. They had many activities in the home for stimulation. The staff worked together well, which was a big advantage since happy workers usually mean happy residents. A disgruntled staff creates a tense atmosphere and sometimes leads to abuse. The residents can sense the unhappiness.

I have also played music in facilities in very small farm communities in Wisconsin. There, I have found, facilities are well-run and staffed by caring people. This is partly because the caregivers and patients are from the same community—neighbors are caring for neighbors. There is plenty of help. People on neighboring farms come in to cook, clean, and visit the residents. Some mend clothes, run errands, and help the residents in various ways. Their attitude is, "We are all in this together—taking care of the elderly is in the best interest of our community." Such a place gives me a very warm fuzzy feeling.

Many large nursing homes have cut back on staff benefits by cutting wages, eliminating higher holiday pay, and cutting back on health benefits. When a facility is short-staffed, it is not likely to be able to fulfill its mission statement. However, in your area the opposite may be true—the small-town facilities may be short-staffed and underfunded, while the larger nursing homes may be well-run with a trained staff.

It is best to be very picky about selecting a care facility. I never had to worry about my mom when she was in the group home I had selected, because the staffers were good, solid people. Remember, your frequent visits will make a difference in the care your loved one receives. Make friends with the caregivers. I would bring treats for the staff. Keep in touch with your loved one, and remain informed of the care plans and changes in care needs as the disease progresses. This will help you be prepared in the event that your loved one requires more care and must be moved to another facility. If you see this coming, you can get on a waiting list early so that you won't be caught with few or no options, or with only bad ones.

Hospice Care

Hospice care differs from curative care. The prime goal of hospice care is to keep the terminal patient emotionally and physically comfortable, taking pain management into consideration. Hospice means care, comfort, and support not only of the patient but also of the family. Many hospice teams will continue to work with the family following the death of a loved one. Counseling can take place to help the family get through the crisis time and to help heal their emotional pain.

A hospice team is made up of physicians, registered nurses, trained volunteers, and sometimes a chaplain or other religious leader, who work to meet the needs of the terminally ill patient and the family. Hospice teams work both in homes and nursing facilities. One of my friends works with hospice. She had watched her mother die of cancer and took the training because she wanted to help other families. It was a healing process for her. She had a beautiful way with the elderly. As a volunteer she was able to make the terminally ill comfortable.

I remember a hospice worker coming to a care facility where I worked as an activity assistant. Ruth, the patient, was a beautiful lady with an outstanding attitude. She was not angry that she had terminal cancer. She was surrounded by her family. The nurse also came daily to visit her. I was allowed to visit her a few minutes a day and I prayed with her at her bedside. To this day, I treasure my memories of this beautiful lady. She asked me to pray with her so God would call her home and take away the mental anguish. She thanked God for having a good life and a wonderful family. God granted her wish after 30 days with hospice care.

It is important to note that an Alzheimer's patient in her last stages can also benefit from hospice care. My Aunt Gene had hospice care in the nursing facility. She became physically sick and lost a lot of weight. Many Alzheimer's patients develop pneumonia and have a hard time bouncing back or lose the ability to swallow food.

To find out about hospice care, check with your physician, local hospital, or religious advisor. Make an appointment with a hospice care group to learn about all the aspects of the program. Call National Hospice Organization, Arlington, VA (703) 243-5900 or (800) 658-

8898. Most insurance companies offer policies with hospice benefits. Hospice care can also be covered by benefits under Medicare and Medicaid—check your insurance policy.

Make sure that the hospice care you choose can meet the patient's needs. If hospice care occurs in the home make sure you have a hospital bed and all the equipment necessary to make your loved one comfortable. Follow the instructions of the hospice professionals and be there for your loved one. It can be a beautiful time for your family and loved one because you have the opportunity to be with them and share their last days.

Preparing for Your Loved One's Final Journey Home

Whether at home or in a care facility, you may want to have hospice care. While working at a care facility I watched the hospice caregivers. They are trained to be with the patient. I saw total dedication and love for the dying person. As an activity director in a care facility, I sometimes stayed after hours to gain experience. Many times, I held a resident's hand as they were dying. Most residents were at peace and were ready to die. Just being there for the person in a quiet manner has a calming effect.

Because I lost my mother to Alzheimer's and then to death, I find serenity in helping others with the disease. It helps take away my pain of having lost my mother. Sitting with the dying is not for everyone. As human beings we all act and react differently. I find it very interesting that most elderly people know when death is near. My mother had a lucid moment when I held her hand and she knew her time was short, despite the Alzheimer's disease. It is very rewarding to me to be able to comfort the dying and help them be at peace.

After my mom's death, I prepared for the funeral service. Because Mom had taken care of funeral arrangements in advance, the funeral director could take charge of that end of it. He already had the names and addresses of our surviving family members. He contacted the church, florist, and newspaper. That all helps take the stress off family members. He also can contact a caterer or restaurant for a lunch after the funeral. Because I was a professional caterer I made the lunch. It was good therapy for me. We only had a few people because Mom had lived to be 89 and had outlived most family members and friends. I had catered my dad's funeral lunch and wanted to do the same for my mom. Whatever you decide to do it should be decided in advance to help the process go smoothly. You also need time to grieve. I did not find time to grieve until a week later. You may need to attend class to help you get through the grieving process. Funeral homes have many pamphlets on death and grieving.

Autopsy

The only way you can confirm that your loved one had Alzheimer's disease is through an autopsy. Any blood relative can order an autopsy. Read your state's statutes in advance and be prepared to order the autopsy. The doctor can examine the brain and confirm the presence of the disease. Make sure the death certificate states that evidence of Alzheimer's was present. Sometimes family members do not want an autopsy performed. One woman was afraid her mother would be "all cut up." Another did not want to spend the money for one.

I was glad that my mom had an autopsy. The doctor had encouraged our family to have it done. And no one could even tell that it had been done.

You can usually get autopsy consent papers from the doctor. It simplifies things a great deal if you put in writing in advance that you wish to have an autopsy performed.

Chapter 7:

Resources

The Alzheimer's Association

The Alzheimer's Association was founded in 1980 with 200 chapters nationwide. The Alzheimer's Association is the largest national voluntary health organization working to conquer this disease. It is a nonprofit organization with programs reaching out to help professionals, trained caregivers, families, friends, and patients, keeping them informed on the latest medical breakthroughs as well as helping them cope with the effects of the disease.

Their motto is "stand by you" and they work very hard to get information out to the public. There are many support groups across the United States that hold meetings each week to reach out to the caregivers. Regional outreach programs sponsored by the Alzheimer's Association are located throughout the United States.

Many funds have been raised for research in hopes for a cure. Each chapter hands out pamphlets with information about the disease, about driving and dementia, and has a library with books and tapes pertaining to the disease. I was very lucky to have the Alzheimer's Association as a ready reference when my mom first was diagnosed.

There are several support groups to help caregivers and professionals. One support leader started a men's group that has been very successful in our area.

Many people are afraid to ask for help or are in denial that their loved one has Alzheimer's. That makes it difficult to help those people.

The Alzheimer's Association has a special support system that will guide you through difficult times. In some cases, staff members and volunteers have taken special training, and in addition have or had a loved one afflicted with AD. In many cases these folks are strong advocates for the elderly and understand what you are going through with your loved one. Experience makes for a good teacher.

I found acceptance that my mother had Alzheimer's and asking how to do what was in her best interest really helped me a lot. Professional advice and follow-through helped me keep my sanity. The Alzheimer's Association chapters across the country have family support groups, help lines, seminars, and books and information to help with all facets of Alzheimer's disease or other forms of dementia.

Some Alzheimer's Association chapters have the following services:

Respite care program:
Provides relief for the caregivers.

Education:
Books and lectures on topics relevant to Alzheimer's disease.

Advocacy:
There are several issues involved with Alzheimer's that require legislation. The Association works on public policy changes in a variety of areas. For example, the Southeastern Wisconsin Alzheimer's Association chapter's advocacy committee meets once every month to address issues. I have been on this committee for the last four years. A team goes to Washington once a year to talk with our political leaders about Alzheimer's issues.

Most Alzheimer's chapters have newsletters, workshops, family support groups, training for how to cope, in-service training, and the medic alert bracelets. Check in with your local Alzheimer's Association chapter to find what services best fit your needs.

The Alzheimer's Association
919 N. Michigan Avenue, Suite 1100
Chicago, Illinois 60611
www.alz.org
(312) 335-8700 or (800) 272-3900 is a 24-hour contact center for the
National Alzheimer Association.

The Alzheimer's Association Memory Walk

The Memory Walk is a time for friends, families, and co-workers to enjoy the day and unite together to fight against the Alzheimer's disease. This walk brings awareness to the heartbreaking disease. The monies go to the Alzheimer's Association chapter in your area to help fund its existing services. The monies also help develop new programs to help meet the needs of families and caregivers, and support a toll-free help line, consultations with family members, an up-to-date resource library, materials, support groups, and a quarterly newsletter. In addition, there are the Safe Return bracelets, a large variety of quality educational programs, and advocating work for legislation that eases the hardship on families. There is also an early-stage patient support group. Each chapter supports research for a cure for Alzheimer's disease. To date, no cure has been found, but researchers say there have been many major breakthroughs.

(Description of Memory Walk courtesy of Alzheimer's Association.)

People walk because they have been touched in some way by this disease. Participants walk alone, in family groups, or in teams, and sign up sponsors to pledge money for each mile walked. I organized a group of members of my parish. When I was working with our assistant pastor on a name for our group, I told him I was envisioning a path and feet walking to find memory. He suggested "Pathfinder for Memory." That is how our team name came to be. We even designed our own logo (see above inset). It is a wonderful day. The Memory Walk is usually the largest fundraiser for the year.

I might also add that all the food and prizes are donated. Local companies underwrite the costs of the walk. Each walker is encouraged to raise a minimum suggested amount found on the form. The checks are to be made to the local Alzheimer's Association chapter.

The Assisted Living Federation of America
103 Eaton Place, Suite 400
Fairfax, VA 22030
Phone: (703) 691-8100 Fax: (703) 691-8106
e-mail: lc@alfa.org

You can e-mail with questions or comments about their website. You can visit their searchable ALFA Online Directory at www.careguide.net.

You can search for assisted living residences by state, county, city, or metropolitan area with interactive maps. You also can get additional listings including information about specific services and programs. Most assisted living facilities try hard to give the resident as much independence and freedom as possible but also give personal care. They work hard to treat the elderly person with dignity. Three meals are provided daily, and medications are dispensed. There are often beauty shop appointments, mail delivery, and many activities.

What is Medicare?

Medicare is a health insurance program for some people with disabilities under 65 years of age, for people 65 years and older, or for people with permanent kidney failure who require dialysis or kidney transplant. Medicare Part A helps pay for skilled nursing facilities, hospice, skilled nursing facilities, and some home health care. Most folks do not have to pay a monthly payment for a premium for Part A because one or both of the spouses paid Medicare taxes while they were working. For help about your Medicare benefits call 1-800-Medicare [(800) 633-4227] or TTY/TDD (for hard of hearing): (877) 486-2048 for hearing and speech impaired. Internet address is www.medicare.gov, then click on "Important Contacts." The Medicare number will also provide you with fiscal intermediary information. In addition you may call your State Health Insurance Assistance Program by using the Medicare number. If you get benefits from the railroad call Railroad Retirement Board at (800) 808-0772.

Ask about the number for your regional home health intermediary information. Each state has a listing. Also at the Medicare number you can get a booklet called *The Guide to Health Insurance for People with Medicare* which is also available on audio tape, in large type, or in Braille.

Part B is supplemental insurance, paid for monthly, to help with doctor's services, outpatient hospital care, and some other medical services when Part A does not cover the bill (for example, Part A does not cover physical and occupational therapists).You can sign up for Part B three months before you turn 65. You can call your local Social Security Office or go in person to sign up. Your premium is taken out of your monthly Social Security check. Make sure that your doctor accepts your Medicare plan.

Co-payment means the part you have to pay that insurance doesn't cover. For example, under a "20/80" plan, you pay 20 percent and the insurance pays 80 percent. It is wise to have a co-pay insurance plan for prescriptions so you will not have to pay the full price for medications. Be sure you stay informed about your benefits—co-payments and expenses covered can change from year to year.

You can also call the Insurance Consumer Helpline in Washington D.C. for more information (800) 942-4242.

What is a Medigap policy?

A Medigap policy is sold by a private insurance company to help fill the gaps in Medicare plan coverage. The Medigap policy must say it is for Medicare Supplement on the first page of the policy. People purchasing Medigap policies after 1990 will have the policy automatically renewed each year provided that the premiums are paid. You must pay your monthly Medicare Part B premium.

If you have financial power of attorney for an elderly person, be sure you study the information so you can best serve the person's needs. My mother had Medicare A and B. The supplemental insurance was a big help. It is very expensive to care for an Alzheimer's patient, so it is wise to be prepared just in case. You will need to use their money on them in their best interest.

Caregiving Tips—a Review

■ Remember that the Alzheimer's patient is in his/her own little world so the caregiver must play along. Basically the Alzheimer's patient lives life in the past. Living in the past makes the person feel more comfortable.

■ It is best not to accuse the person of lying—because the person lives in the past, their understanding of the world is different. Due to their lack of memory the AD person just fills in from the past experiences, they are not necessarily reflecting what is real. Help the person feel secure and get into their world to alleviate the AD person's fears or loss of security.

■ Use distraction when the AD person becomes agitated. Change the subject and then go back to the topic later, when the patient is calmer. Remember the short-term memory is gone, so use that to your advantage with distraction and change the subject.

■ Don't take remarks to heart. One patient I worked with said, "I like your dress. It is ugly." I did not get upset. She did not understand her words any longer. In addition a confused person often misjudges situations. Some become overly suspicious. My mom was very suspicious that the banker was stealing her Social Security check when he did not do any such thing. She also lost her good manners. I always had to pinch myself and just say, this is not my mother anymore. I accepted the things I could not change but still continued to love her unconditionally.

■ Follow a simple, set routine. Keep the patient calm by going with the flow and do not argue or reason with the patient. It does not work. The caregiver and patient both get upset and there is a lot of trouble when this happens. Sometimes abuse occurs between the caregiver and the AD patient. Remember that someone with AD can become very combative when frightened. Change can be very upsetting. Avoid loud noise and a great deal of excitement.

■ Constant encouragement and clues are needed to help the AD person perform activities of the day. My mom could dress herself if I laid out her clothes in order.

■ Demonstrate with love and patience how to do a task in order to get the AD person to follow.

■ Praise the person's accomplishments.

■ The caregiver should never appear angry, hostile, or frustrated with the AD person. Try to anticipate problems and avoid them before they happen.

■ Each day work with the AD person to get proper exercise and diet. Just make it part of your routine.

■ The AD person generally loses track of time, date, day, month, and year. Mom wore a watch all her life. I got her a watch with big numbers and she pretended she knew the time. That was just fine with me. She enjoyed wearing it and reading the time of day in her own little world on her time.

■ Do not think that a person can understand and act on messages whether written or verbal.

■ Break down directions into simple steps. Give the person plenty of time to follow through. Do not rush or hurry them.

■ Encourage persons to get involved in activities. Live for the moment and smile and laugh with them, for laughter will keep you sane. Above all give as many pleasures as possible to the AD person during their day. It is the little things that count. To know the person, is to serve the person well.

■ Bear in mind that the person has lost the ability to make good judgments in most situations as far as being safe or unsafe. You, the caregiver, must evaluate each situation and keep them out of danger. You are the protector. I found it is hard job because you want to protect them but still want them to enjoy life. I had to work hard at finding a balance.

■ Remember, the AD person's peripheral vision is very different from ours. Don't walk up from behind them unannounced. They may become frightened and very agitated.

Books and Videotapes

The best book I have read on Alzheimer's is *The Validation Breakthrough: Simple Techniques for Communicating With People With Alzheimer's-type Dementia*, by Naomi Feil. I have read this book several times and still find it helpful. I have applied the techniques Feil recommends and have found that they work beautifully. The validation techniques this book describes can be used by anyone who works with people with dementia: lawyers, doctors, nurses, judges, social workers, friends, and family members.

I also recommend two audio tapes by Feil titled "Communicating with the Alzheimer's-type Population" and "Looking for Yesterday." These tapes help caregivers understand how to get into the world of the Alzheimer's patient.

The first tape describes ways caregivers can use validation to help the person feel more comfortable and to give them dignity. The second describes how Alzheimer's patients become time-confused and begin recreating events that happened long ago in their lives.

Feil describes how "reality orientation" (correcting or contradicting the person when they are irrational) serves only to frustrate and anger the person. Convincing a person that she is confused or wrong is impossible. Arguing with a person with dementia is futile. Instead, become a reporter and ask questions using non-threatening words, and don't hold them accountable for their actions.

I also recommend *Partial View* by Cary Smith Henderson. This book is Henderson's first-person account of living with Alzheimer's. He was a college professor, and started writing this book when he was first diagnosed; his daughter helped him finish writing in the later stages. The author told his feelings and he wished that people would not treat him so differently. He recognized that he could not do the things he used to do and relied heavily on his wife to get through his days.

He tells of looking up the flights of stairs in his home and worrying about how he was going to place his feet to get up the stairs.

His book helped me better understand why my mother "shadowed" me. (She would walk behind me, watching where my feet were placed, so she could follow.)

You may want to read *Aging with Grace* by Dr. David Snowdon. He studied nuns living in a convent for several years, and gained important insights into Alzheimer's disease and the aging process. One of his conclusions from his study is that the more intellectually active you remain in your life, the better chance you have to avoid dementia. *Time* magazine ran a cover story on his study on May 14, 2001.

Other Sources of Help

Some communities have senior counseling centers that charge for their services and counsel families with special needs and problems such as families touched by the Alzheimer's disease. It helps to know that you are not alone. These centers are often located at a hospital as part of their services.

In the Milwaukee area you can call the Wisconsin Geriatric Education Center at (414) 288-3712. This center has many caregiver tips and also offers help.

Other organizations such as the Department of Aging will give out information on services within your community and also will investigate any elder abuse. Home health organizations and visiting nurses can also help you and your loved one. Get help before you become burned out.

Some caregivers have shared with me that the parent would not let the help in. My mother did not want to let the help in, either. I stayed with Mom and the helper for a half-hour or so. We got Mom involved in an activity and then I disappeared to swim and regroup. Each time, I would only be gone one to two hours. It helped my disposition greatly.

My Personal Crusade

When my mother first was diagnosed with Alzheimer's, I told her I was writing a cookbook and I planned to dedicate it to her. She said, "Save me a copy." Sadly, Mom died before the book was finished. I saved the first copy and wrote her a love note for when I see her in heaven. The name of the book is *Picnics: Catering on the Move*. I am selling it to help raise funds for the Alzheimer's Association and to reach out and help others. A portion of the profit is going to the Alzheimer's Association for educational programs for caregivers and training.

As I travel throughout the United States, I try to get the word out that there is help for caregivers and loved ones dealing with Alzheimer's patients. You can purchase copies of my book and can read an article that tells my story at www.bookzone.com, under "picnics" or "Pat Nekola." I want to keep my mother's memory alive. She was a great cook. In fact, those were happy times for her and me. I use my cookbook as a tool to help increase awareness of this disease when I am doing book signings or talking to groups.

From the time I was a young girl, my mother and I used to make 100 pounds of potato salad together on Dignus Day (the day after Easter) every year. Making this dish was a memory I could share with my mother when she had Alzheimer's. I included my mother's potato salad recipe in my *Picnics* book in her honor.

So many people have come forward to share their stories and the pain of losing their loved ones to Alzheimer's. It has been a joy to share and bond with family members because of the pain endured in their loss.

While at a book signing in the Chicago area, a gentleman came up to me and said, "I am glad you are here. I lost my dad to Alzheimer's. I visited him regularly and took him to McDonald's for coffee. That was his daily ritual after his retirement. One day as we sat down for coffee, Dad pulled out two cards. One was from my daughter and the other was in Dad's garbled handwriting, thanking the nice lady for sending him such a lovely card. He told me he had no idea who this lady was who'd sent him a card, but he wanted to thank her for remembering him." The gentleman's heart was broken that his father didn't recognize his own granddaughter's name, but he simply told his dad that he'd find out who the nice lady was and get the card to her. He kept the card. I told the gentleman to frame that special card, and to hold those memories in his heart to carry with him forever.

Once when I was at a book signing in a suburb of Chicago, a woman came to me and said, "I lost my husband to Alzheimer's when he was 40, and then to death when he was 47." I threw my arms around her and held her tight as the tears streamed down her cheeks. I did not have to say a word. My hug and silence was a heartfelt moment for both of us.

Another time, a young man of 24 came to me and said, "I lost my grandmother to Alzheimer's. At first I was so angry. After feeling terrible for a couple of months, I made up my mind that this beautiful lady was still my grandmother even though she was not the same.

I began to visit her frequently. I took a pad of paper and my pen along each time. I documented many of our conversations after our visits. I learned all about her childhood and her memories of the past. "Now I know why she had Alzheimer's," he said. "I can now tell the beautiful stories about my grandmother to my children and their children. It is a beautiful treasure." I put my hand out and squeezed his hand.

"How wonderful," I said. He hugged me.

These memories carry a person through sad moments. These times with family members who have dealt with the pain of Alzheimer's disease are my treasures that I carry through my daily living.

Knowing what to do and how to respond to the AD person with wisdom and love is a big factor in serving the person with kindness. As I mentioned before, I found that laughter can help the caregiver stay calm. Finally I accepted the things I could not change and worked diligently to treat Mom with dignity, giving her some pleasures of the day to make her happy in her own little world.

It became a big treasure. Her happy responses gave me happiness in return. I learned to live for the moment with my mother. I did not have any high expectations. I accepted what came my way. Many prayers helped me get through the difficult times. God has become an invisible hug in my daily life which has helped conquer what I thought was the impossible mission.

Please do your homework, get help, and follow through to serve with love your relative, friend, or resident with Alzheimer's.

Chapter 8:

The Role of an Activity Director in a Care Facility

The recreational therapy staff members should be very people-oriented and enjoy working with the elder population. An activity director must have high energy and a caring heart, patience, and the education and training to understand the needs of the Alzheimer's patient.

In a way, a care facility is a melting pot. You work with all kinds of people from every walk of life, the majority of whom are women. In this respect, the care facility in which I worked was typical: of 100 residents, only ten were men. It is important to respect the values of the residents' generation. I always stress the importance of treating the elderly with dignity. I work with residents from a Christian (mostly Catholic) background; therefore I've included a number of hymns and religious activities. As a caregiver in a facility, you should determine the religious backgrounds of your patients and help them fulfill their religious needs.

Activities staff members are very important because they keep the residents active and happy. A good activity director and department make the care facility come to life. He/she gets the other staff members and the residents' families involved. A monthly newsletter and some family activities such as Grandparent's Day, a family picnic, and a fall festival give the families an opportunity to connect with their loved ones and build support for the activities department.

As an activity director, I sent monthly newsletters to each resident's family's home to keep them informed of daily activities. I also delivered the calendar personally to each resident, inviting them to participate. When they came, we thanked them, and praised them for coming. When residents were unwilling to leave their rooms, I called family members and encouraged them to visit. The families' involvement was a great boost to our program; it became a team effort. Some brought extra treats or made donations for ice cream.

The ability to stay involved in the community gives the residents a sense of pride and belonging. Once, the residents at our care facility made and sold 50 apple pies and donated the profits to a women's center and heart foundation. Another time, they presented handmade pictures to children at the Ronald McDonald House. These things made the residents feel good and useful. One woman in the second stage of Alzheimer's amazed me. She could not remember how to peel apples, but she could quarter, core, and slice an apple very well. Being a part of this worthy project made her feel important, and she enjoyed socializing with the others. The repetition of slicing apples was good for her. Another woman could peel an apple without breaking the peel. (If you think that is easy, try it sometime.)

The activities are only a small part of the picture. An activity director oversees the activity staff, sets up and maintains a detailed care plan, documents daily activity attendance, maintains progress notes, and is involved with care plans for each resident. At care plan meetings, family members attend to discuss progress, improvements, and concerns. While some families don't bother to show up, there are many concerned families that don't miss a care plan meeting. Charts are set up for each resident, and care plans are set up by each department. Every three months a care conference is arranged with the family, and staff on the progress of the resident. The meeting includes the head nurse, activity director, physical therapist, social worker, the family, and the resident (if the resident is incapacitated or incompetent, the family often requests that he/she not attend). Each department keeps track of each resident's well-being. Examples of an activity progress note and health care center therapeutic recreation assessment can be found starting on page 113.

Also included is an activities RAP (Resident Assessment Protocol) module example, which helps the staff keep track of the resident's status. A MDS sheet (Minimum Data Status) is also kept on each resident. These show the amount of their participation in activities, and are reviewed quarterly by the staff.

The activity department must formulate information under the following categories:
- Medical problems/physical conditions.
- Emotional/intellectual state.
- Perception of problems.
- Placement in correct type of facility (assisted living, etc.).
- Background.
- Performance and habits.

The more an activities staff learns about the residents the better they can serve them.

There are progress notes and update sheets to measure the resident's participation, socialization, and behaviors. A review of goals and plans and new goals and plans are usually listed on a separate sheet of paper.

The activity director and staff could not understand why a patient's behavior was improper. The staff would bring this gentleman to the activity area and he would kneel on the floor and scratch the floor with his fingernails. The floor was terrazzo.

The activity director did her homework and delved into his past, she found he had been a school custodian and it was his job to scrape the gum off the lunchroom floor. (The lunchroom had a terrazzo floor.) Once the activity director found this out she gave him a broom and he swept the area an hour every day. She also covered the floor where he sat in the activity room so the terrazzo didn't show and that solved the behavioral problem.

Note: *When formulating care plans you must consider the entire picture from activities, the approach, scheduling appropriate social activities, where the activity is taking place, special needs and limitations, guidance and supervision, resources and responsibility of the activity person(s). The staff is often inundated with paperwork, and it becomes a juggling act to complete the paperwork required by the government and to spend time with the residents. Every department must keep records. Most workers would rather spend their time with the residents, but paperwork is part of the job.*

One of the reasons I left my job at the care facility was the paperwork. I preferred spending my time with the residents. I find that working as a freelance music therapist is better for me. It allows me to mingle with residents and dedicate my time to them, and I have no paper-work or documentation to do.

Certification Information

If you wish to become a certified activity director, call the National Certification Council of Activity Professionals at (757) 552-0653 from 9 a.m. to 5 p.m. EST, or visit their website: www.nccap.org. Local nursing homes can also tell you where training is available in your area for you to become certified. There are two classes in activity management (basic and advanced). The basic course covers core planning, documentation, group process, re-motivation, music, crafts, validation, reminiscence, sensory activities, and special events. The advanced course covers activity program systems, administrative practice, time management, communication, and community relations.

Some of the documents directors fill out and refer to are: resident's daily activity report, recreational therapy department progress notes, activity progress notes, resident activity attendance sheet.

Therapeutic Recreation Department
Assessment/General Data, History

Name: _____

Diagnosis: _____

Mental status: _____

Diet/alcohol restriction: _____

Previous lifestyle/interests: _____

_____

_____

Educational and occupational background: _____

_____

_____

_____

Activities/interests:

❏ cards/games	❏ crafts/arts	❏ exercise/sports
❏ music	❏ reading/writing	❏ baking
❏ sing-a-long	❏ current events	❏ gardening
❏ special events	❏ spiritual/religion	❏ trips
❏ shopping	❏ outdoors	❏ walks
❏ TV	❏ bingo	❏ pet therapy
❏ community involvement	❏ hobbies	❏ travel
❏ meal activities (luncheons/breakfasts)		

Mental functioning (check all that apply):

❏ aware of person	❏ aware of place
❏ aware of time	❏ aware of self
❏ independently makes decisions	❏ unable to make decisions
❏ needs help to make decisions	❏ unable to assess
❏ poor short-term memory	❏ good short-term memory
❏ good long-term memory	
❏ poor attention span (< 5 minutes)	
❏ moderate attention span (5-10 minutes)	
❏ good attention span (>10 minutes)	
❏ able to make needs known	

Social functioning:

❏ initiates conversation   ❏ responds to questions

❏ interacts with peers   ❏ interacts with staff

❏ prefers to be alone   ❏ prefers small groups

❏ prefers to be with one other person   ❏ prefers large groups

❏ eats all meals in room

❏ eats meals in dining room

❏ unable to assess

Perspective on resident recreational involvement:

❏ unable to communicate interests/needs

❏ denies need for recreational outlets

❏ ambivalent regarding need for recreational activities

❏ recognizes need for recreational outlets

Recommended therapeutic intervention:

❏ 1:1 intervention required

❏ leisure education required

❏ willing to become involved in formal programs but will require assistance to attend and participate

❏ assistance in planning and obtaining materials required

Additional comments:

_____

_____

_____

_____

_____

_____

Current interests (describe how the resident enjoys spending current leisure time, including level of involvement in community, church, and family. Also include any hobbies, sports, or individual pursuits.):

The resident's expectation of how his/her day will be spent here:

Physical functioning:

Hearing:

❑   hears within normal tones

❑   uses hearing aid (1 or 2)

❑   speaker must face resident when speaking

❑   speak directly into ear (right or left)

❑   either ear

❑   unable to assess

Speech:

❏ clear   ❏ slurred   ❏ soft spoken

❏ aphasia (expressive, receptive)

❏ needs to write message   ❏ unable to assess

Vision:

❏ adequate with glasses

❏ adequate without glasses

❏ glasses for reading

❏ blurred

❏ unable to see

❏ unable to assess

Mobility/tolerance:

❏ limited time up (a.m., afternoons, p.m.)

❏ up most of the day

❏ up evenings

❏ needs wheelchair

❏ needs walker

❏ ambulates independently

❏ geri chair

❏ bed rest

❏ is able to complete projects independently or with reminders

❏ needs assistance to complete projects

ACTIVITIES RAP (Resident Activity Protocol) MODULE

Resident's name:

Problems to be considered as activity plan is developed (Answer all with yes, no or n/a):

Cognitive:

Do available activities correspond to resident's lifetime values, attitudes, and expectations?

Does resident consider "leisure activities" a waste of time?

Would resident benefit from activities requiring lower activity levels?

Does resident have cognitive/functional deficits that either reduce options or preclude involvement in all/most activities that would otherwise be of interest?

Treatment and conditions:

Is resident suffering from an acute health problem?

Is resident hindered because of embarrassment/unease due to presence of health-related equipment?

Has resident recently recovered from an illness?

Has an illness left resident with some disability?

Does resident possess skills or have the capacity to learn new skills sufficient to permit greater involvement?

Is there substantial reason to believe resident cannot tolerate or would be harmed by increased activity level?

Does resident retain any desire to learn or master a specific new activity?

Does the facility's environment hamper involvement in activities for this resident?

Has there been a lack of provided activities indicated as preferred?

Environmental factors:

Are current activity levels affected by the season of the year or the nature of the weather during the M.D.'s assessment period?

Can resident choose to participate in or to create an activity?

Has a staff person who has been instrumental in involving the resident in activities left the facility/been reassigned?

Is a new member in a group activity viewed by resident as taking over?

Has another resident who was a leader on the unit died or left the unit?

Is the resident shy/unable to make new friends?

Does resident's expression of dissatisfaction with fellow residents indicate resident does not want to be part of activities group?

Does resident have a cardiac problem or other disease that might suggest a need to slow down?

Diagnosis/medication:

Is resident on medication that would limit or interfere with participation in activities?

Does the resident participate in activity program to the extent of physical/cognitive ability or limitations?

Would the quality of this resident's life be enhanced by a revised activity plan?

Care plan decision:

❏ proceed   ❏ do not proceed

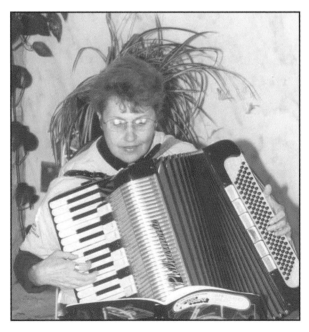

Volunteer
Pat Nekola playing her accordian at the Memory Walk.

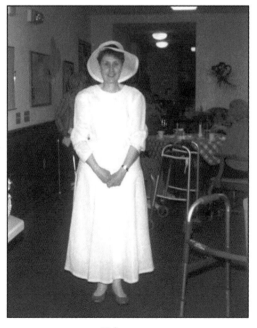

Volunteer
Pat Nekola volunteering a friendly visit to the facility where her mother resided.

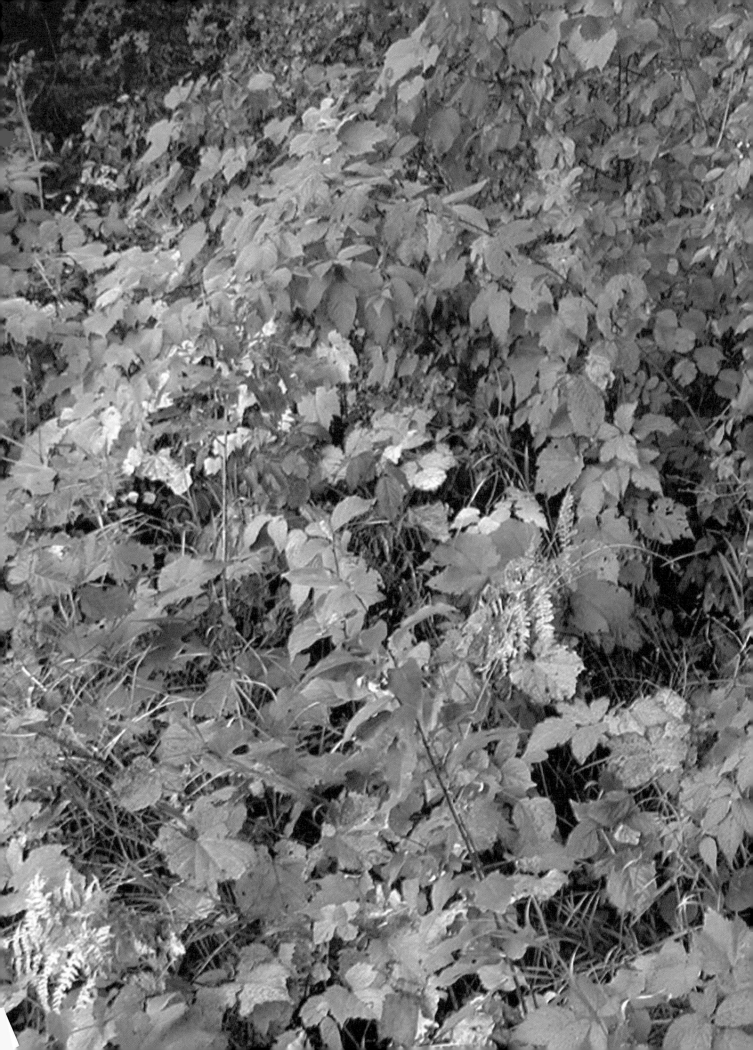

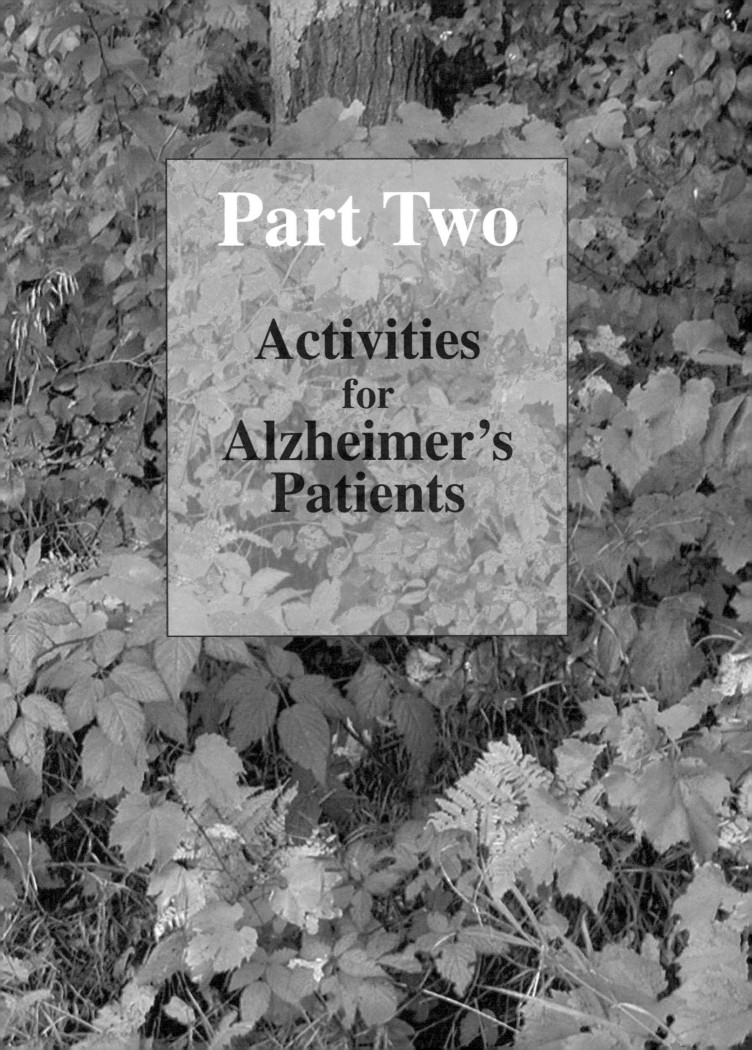

Part Two

Activities
for
Alzheimer's
Patients

Chapter 9:

JANUARY

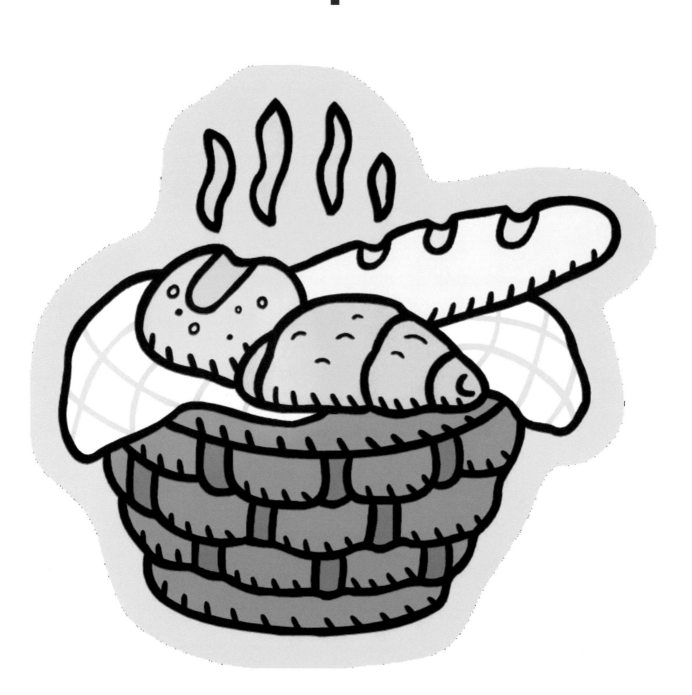

Heart and Hands

As I worked on putting together my programs, I kept in mind it is the little things that count for the elderly. They are big to them and very meaningful. The things we take for granted are precious to them. I wanted to make them feel comfortable in a group. I found residents respond not to the material alone but to how it is presented to them in a safe and comfortable environment. Making the person feel wanted as a part of the group is a must. How the activity person presents him- or herself can make or break the success of the program. I always make a point to greet and welcome everyone in the group. Praising residents for coming and recognizing them for participation often helps too. There was a resident that came for activities each week. She said very little but I could tell by her facial expressions she was benefiting from the program. On this special day I asked her how she was feeling. She said she didn't feel well. I replied, "I sure hope you will feel better soon. I am just happy you came today. I would miss you and be lonesome for you if you did not come." She extended her hand to me for the first time in nine months of the program. I gladly held her hand.

She said, "And I thank you for being here for me."

It meant a lot to me. It only confirmed the importance of having a loving heart and hand. I also knew she felt comfortable extending her hand to me. Those are the perks that continue to spur me on to do this work.

Thought Process, First-stage to the Beginning of Second-stage Alzheimer's

As I observed care facility residents, I saw how Alzheimer's affected their thought processes, so I put together exercises. I used objects to create hands-on activities. Visual aids are very important to help the thought process. We talked about these activities with the residents, breaking them down into easy steps. The residents can actually perform some of these activities, like folding laundry; others should just be discussed. All activities should be closely supervised.

Doing laundry:
1. Gather clothes.
2. Sort clothes.
3. Put sorted clothes into the washer.
4. Add soap (be aware that some residents may try to eat the soap, so watch them carefully).
5. Start the washer on proper cycle.

Yard work:
1. Mow the lawn.
2. Rake leaves (I actually brought in leaves and a rake to the facility. I spread the leaves on the floor and we raked them up. The residents enjoyed looking at the colors of the leaves, listening to them rustle, and breathing in their scent).
3. Dig dirt.
4. Plant flowers.
5. Water flowers.
6. Pick flowers.
7. Smell flowers.

Make stew (I made stew with my mother and others. We all enjoyed the stew for lunch):
1. Peel carrots and potatoes.
2. Cut vegetables.
3. Brown the stew meat.
4. Season the stew.
5. Stir the pot.
6. Taste the stew.

Sewing on buttons:
1. Cut a length of thread.
2. Thread the needle.
3. Knot the thread.
4. Sew on the button.

Taking care of a baby:
1. Rock the baby (my mom enjoyed rocking a baby).
2. Change the diaper.
3. Feed the baby.
4. Burp the baby.
5. Walk the baby in a stroller.

The above are thought process exercises to help the Alzheimer's residents organize the steps of tasks. I actually do some of these exercises with the residents. Remember that they must be supervised closely if they're actually participating in one of these exercises. Select one topic, such as making stew (see page 135 for recipe), and go through the motions with the residents. Actually peel the carrots and potatoes. My mother and I had fun with this exercise. She peeled the carrots and potatoes while I browned the stew meat. We made enough stew for the entire group home. Mom did quantity cooking all her life. This was a very good exercise for her. The baby exercise is very good for the ladies. Both men and women enjoyed the yard work exercise.

Sensory Activity: Perfumes and Creams

Supplies needed:

10-20 tongue depressors

A variety of perfumes and creams in scents such as almond, peach, vanilla, lilac, and lavender. **Note:** *Many times free samples can be picked up at local stores in the area for this exercise.*

On each tongue depressor spray one variety of perfume or spread a dab of one cream. Walk around and let each resident enjoy the good smells. Offer to let the resident select a perfume or scented cream. Some will decline while others will want to use some perfume. Using a clean tongue depressor every time, place cream on the resident's hand and let the resident rub their hands if they can; help others that cannot. If their expressions and motions reject this exercise, stop immediately. I have found that most residents enjoy the creams. Many residents also like talcum powder. Keep in mind that the resident has a right to make a choice.

It is interesting to see facial expressions and comments with raising of eyebrows when they are sniffing, saying mm-m-m! One 100-year-old lady said, "I love perfume. I feel so good when I wear perfume. You know, if you wear a good smelling perfume you may attract a man." The residents' memories are triggered by the smells.

In addition I had two pungent smells such as vinegar and rubbing alcohol. The residents could tell the difference between sweet and pungent smells.

After the exercise I played several Broadway songs with the residents:

"Get Me to the Church on Time"

"Edelweiss"

"I'm Going to Wash That Man Right Out of My Hair"

"Some Enchanted Evening"

"If I Could Write a Book"

"The Sound of Music"

"Oh What a Beautiful Morning"

"On the Street Where You Live"

"Maria"

"My Favorite Things"

Note: *The residents especially like to hear the tunes from "The Sound of Music."*

Bingo for the Early-stage Alzheimer's Resident

This is for a small group (6-8 people) unless you have a lot of help to coordinate the project.

Supplies needed:

Bingo tally

Bingo cards

Chips to cover the cards

Note: *Laminate the bingo tally and cards.*

Sit with the residents and see if they recognize some of the numbers. Even if they can only pick out a few, it is worth their time. Help the residents cover the cards and say "bingo" as needed. They can win a small prize. Play only two sets of three games. As the disease progresses, the residents may lose interest in playing. The lower numbers may be less confusing and more readily identified than higher numbers, but not in every case. Just play it by ear and

BINGO TALLY

1	2	3	4	5
6	7	8	9	10
11	12	13	14	15

2	6	10
4	7	11
5	9	14

3	6	11
4	8	12
5	10	14

3	6	10
4	9	12
5	10	14

3	6	10
4	8	12
5	9	14

2	6	11
3	7	13
4	9	14

adjust to meet the residents' needs.

One resident who had been a math teacher for 35 years and could still recognize numbers, even in the third stage of Alzheimer's. My mom, in the second stage of Alzheimer's, could still recognize the numbers on the bingo cards. Usually the group home played bingo at night after dinner. She loved to show me the prizes she'd won. She gave me a pair of hot pink gloves from the bingo game. I still have those gloves as a memento. Stuffed animals are very popular prizes. As the disease progresses into the end of the third and beginning of the fourth stages, the residents lose interest in the game and prizes. We took Aunt Gene to regular bingo even though she could no longer read the numbers. We sat with her and one time helped her win a banana for a prize. She enjoyed the activity and the banana. It was good to get her out of her room too. You can make up your own Bingo numbers and use the previous pages of sample sheets as a guide.

Martin Luther King Day

In January we celebrate Martin Luther King Day. I went to the library for the book *I Have A Dream*, which I found in the children's section. There are many beautiful colored pictures that tell the story of Dr. Martin Luther King Jr. I made color copies of the pictures and also the speech. I made up two bulletin boards with the pictures and story. I took the time to tell the story of the life of Dr. Martin Luther King Jr.

Martin Luther King Jr. was born in 1929 and died in 1968. He was a minister and a brilliant, highly-educated man. He was one of the greatest leaders in the civil rights movement, which he saw as an opportunity for all races to unite as brothers and sisters to work together. Segregation and discrimination were prevalent in early America. Slavery was practiced in the South. Many slaves escaped and traveled to Northern states where they were treated better. Some of the freed slaves helped other slaves to freedom. Today African-Americans have the same rights and freedoms as whites. However, even today there are problems with discrimination.

Martin Luther King gave his famous "I Have a Dream" speech in Washington, D.C., by the Washington Monument during an event that made history as the greatest demonstration for freedom in our nation. He was assassinated at the age of 39. He knew he might be assassinated; he was aware of the threats to his life. But it did not stop him from doing his work, for he had strong convictions.

It is people who are willing to make changes for the enrichment of other folks' lives that make the difference. When you have a dream, you make it happen with effort and stick-to-it-iveness.

For the party, I covered the table with patriotic material with an American flag design. I placed a rocket centerpiece with two large bulletin boards with pictures from the children's book *I Have a Dream* and a picture of Dr. Martin Luther King Jr. I also had American flags in stands. I decorated three patriotic wishing wells and one large colorful map of the United States. I asked the residents if they had had a dream. One was alert enough to say, "Yes, I wanted to get married and have a family." I asked if her dream had come true. She said yes. I was amazed that very few people had dreams. As I walked around the room, most had wishes. Some wished they could have candy or favorite food. Others wished for visitors or lots of money. I played all the patriotic songs and this higher functioning group could sing the songs and hymns and clap with the music. Some waved the American flags and played rhythmic instruments. We served cake and punch.

I repeated this activity later that afternoon for the lower functioning residents. I could only go into minor detail. I saw some with "sundowning" problems (some residents get upset or agitated late in the day). So I put the pictures and decorations up and I played 50 minutes of patriotic songs. I basically talked to them and fussed over the residents as I played music and managed to tell some of the story of Dr. Martin Luther King Jr. It is very important to adjust to the abilities of your audience. The music was good for this group. A handful could wave the American flag and hum but most could not sing the songs. That is perfectly all right for they enjoyed the music.

Mom's Old-Fashioned Beef Stew

Yield: 20 servings

$1/4$ cup margarine

4 pounds beef stew meat cut into 1-inch cubes

2 bay leaves

2 medium onions, peeled and diced

2 cups diced celery

10 medium potatoes, peeled, cut into small chunks

10 medium carrots, peeled, cut into sticks

3 cups canned tomatoes, drained, diced

3 tablespoons beef granules

6 cups hot water

2 teaspoons Worcestershire sauce

1 tablespoon A-1 steak sauce

To thicken stew later:

1 cup water

3 tablespoons cornstarch

Few drops caramel color

Melt margarine in large skillet over medium-high heat. Brown the meat in batches. Place in a large full-size steam table pan or Dutch oven. Add bay leaves, onions, celery, potatoes, carrots, and tomatoes. Dissolve beef granules in 6 cups of hot water. Add to meat and vegetable mixture. Add Worcestershire sauce and A-1 steak sauce to mixture and stir. Cover and bake in oven at 275 degrees for 3-4 hours or until meat and vegetables are very tender. Remove bay leaves. Whisk cornstarch into 1 cup water. Stir gradually into the beef stew until thickened. Add few drops of caramel color to finished product to give a golden brown color. Do not add too much caramel color or the stew will turn very dark.

Chapter 10:

FEBRUARY

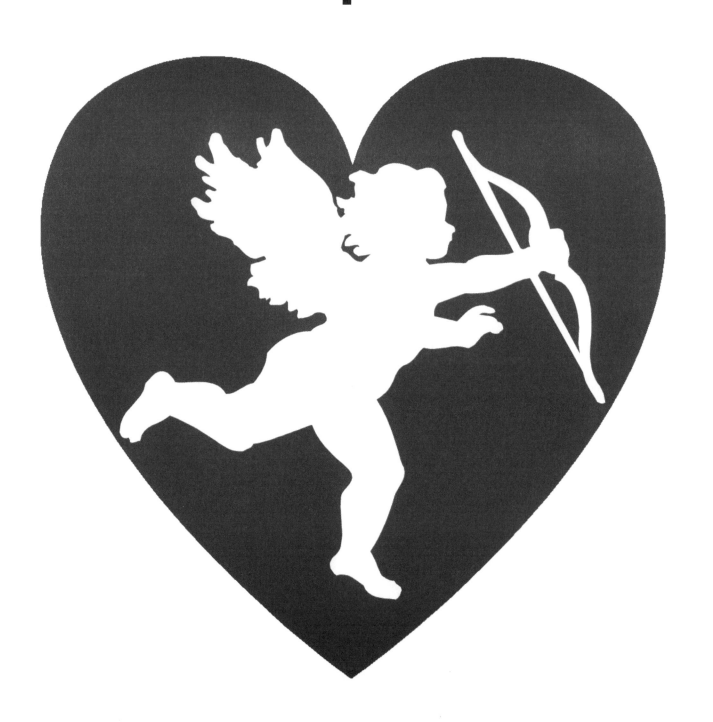

Heart Cookie Cutter Exercise

(for lower functioning Alzheimer's residents)

Supplies needed:

6 heart-shaped cookie cutters in graduated sizes.

The heart cookie cutters should be easy for the resident to grasp.

Drawings of hearts in sizes to match cookie cutters.

Work with one or two low-functioning residents to help them with the various sized hearts. Get the resident to nestle the hearts from the smallest to largest. Next start with the largest heart and nestle the remaining five hearts to the smallest. If the resident cannot comprehend how to nestle all six at once, try two at a time.

In addition you can try to have the resident match the size of the heart cookie cutter to the hearts drawn on the sheet. Always encourage the resident; do not criticize him/her if the task is too difficult. Continue to try various techniques until the resident can accomplish just the smallest task. Praise the resident for his/her accomplishments. If there are too many shapes cover four of the hearts and leave the two hearts showing. Give the resident the two matching cookie cutters and ask which heart should be placed on the paper to match the drawn heart.

If the resident can even remember a little for just a second it makes them feel good, and they enjoy the attention. Do not feel badly if the resident loses interest. A short attention span is very common as the disease progresses.

Valentine's Day heart pins

Supplies needed:
Plastic placemat (preferably pink or red).
Miscellaneous buttons.
Scraps of lace.
Jewelry pin for back of pin.
Craft glue.

Cut heart shapes out of the placemat. The residents can decorate the hearts by gluing buttons and lace on the heart. Glue a pin on the back of the heart and let dry. The residents can wear their pins for Valentine's Day. Some residents will need assistance with this project because they can't pick up the buttons or squeeze the glue bottle. Use small bottles of glue for easy handling. Some may not be able to follow directions. Give one-step directions and assist as necessary. I can't stress enough that patience and your sincere love and kindness are a must when working with lower functioning residents.

Questions Designed with Heart Patterns

Exercise can take 15-20 minutes depending on attention span.

Cut six different-sized hearts out of red paper; or cut them out of white paper and let the residents color them red; some people will enjoy coloring.

What color is the heart? Place the largest red heart on the paper to match the size on the paper. Place the smallest red heart on the paper. Count how many hearts are white on the paper. Touch the smallest heart. How many small hearts are on the paper? Touch the largest heart. Touch the medium size heart. Touch the second smallest heart.

Love Songs

For the low-functioning residents I spent an hour playing songs about hearts and love. I also talked to them about the meaning of the words. I was able to get a few responses. I also played a tape with waltzes and danced with some of the residents in their wheelchairs and geri chairs. It exercises their arm muscles. I held their hands and then gave them gentle hugs. I enjoyed seeing their responses. I also consider the residents that cannot respond or have any expression on their faces. A couple drew a blank but still held my hand.

During the week of Valentine's Day, songs with heart and love themes stimulated the residents and gave them joy for the hour. There are many songs with heart and love themes. Music touches the Alzheimer's patient's heart. It is a wonderful way to get into their world and jog their memories, especially about love. It appeals to the resident's emotions.

"Let Me Call You Sweetheart"
"Be Careful It's my Heart"
"I Poured My Heart Into a Song"
"Cheek to Cheek"
"Coquette"
"Heartaches by the Number"
"We Shall Overcome Some Day"
"May the Good Lord Bless and Keep You"
"My Heart Belongs to Daddy"
"Smile"
"Wonderful, Wonderful"
"San Antonio Rose"
"The Way You Look Tonight"
"I've Got You Under My Skin"
"Chinatown, My Chinatown"
"I Poured My Heart Into a Song"
"Heart of My Heart"
"You Gotta Have Heart"
"Always"
"Because I Love You"

"Blue Skies"
"Fools Fall in Love"
"True Love"
"Love Can Make You Happy"
"Because"
"I Love You Truly"
"When I Fall in Love"
"Love Is in the Air"
"Why Do I Love You?"
"Anniversary Waltz"
"How Deep Is Your Love?"
"Let's Fall in Love"
"Endless Love"
"Ich Leibe Dich (I Love Thee)"
"I've Got My Love to Keep Me Warm"
"Wunderbar"
"The Best Things in Life Are Free"
"Sugar Time"
"That's Amorè"

Kindness, love, and caring is very important to preserve the patient's dignity and let them live for the moment. As they share their memories with me I receive joy. The more I learn about them, the more I can help them live a full life. I appreciate the little things as I watch their frail minds and bodies regress. They accept my kindness and I accept their smiles and laugh with them. I readily forgive any offensive words for many do not understand what they are saying nor will they remember later. Even though some cannot put logical sentences together any longer it is my pleasure to be a gracious listener.

Rhubarb Pie

As I studied residents' backgrounds, I learned that many of them had had gardens. Many grew up in the Depression, and the garden was a way of putting food on the table. My mom talked to me many times about the Depression. The Depression days stuck in her mind as they do for many elderly folks.

Rhubarb grows very readily and so my grandma always made rhubarb sauces, jams, and pies. We all liked her rhubarb pie made with her strawberry jam. It smelled so good when it was freshly baked. She made a lard crust which we no longer do. I have modified Grandma's rhubarb pie recipe for the Alzheimer's resident.

I like to get out the ingredients and talk about them. Some residents recall the farm eggs and going to the chicken coop for eggs each day, while others remember growing the rhubarb. Seeing and smelling really jogs the memory.

Note: The residents enjoy packing the crumbs into the pie pan. It is like packing sand. They like taking turns stirring the filling. The smells of the pie baking stimulates their olfactory senses. It is fun to see their reactions to the good smells.

Granny's Rhubarb Pie

Yield: One 10-inch pie

Crust

2	cups graham cracker crumbs
$1/2$	cup sugar
$3/4$	cup margarine, melted

Filling

1	package (20 ounces) quick-frozen rhubarb pieces
$3/4$	cup sugar
2	cups strawberry jam
2	eggs
1	container (16 ounces) whipped topping
	Sliced fresh strawberries, for garnish

Preheat oven to 350 degrees. In a medium bowl, stir together graham cracker crumbs, sugar, and margarine. Press into the bottom and up the sides of a 10-inch pie pan. Bake crust for 4-5 minutes to set.

For filling, squeeze excess water out of rhubarb. In a bowl, stir sugar into the rhubarb. In a large bowl, stir the strawberry jam and eggs together. Stir rhubarb into the strawberry jam-egg mixture, blending well. Pour into the piecrust. Bake for 20 minutes. Cool. Top with whipped topping and fresh strawberry slices. Serve chilled. Garnish with fresh mint leaves (optional).

A Tribute to Aunt Gene

While driving home from a care facility I began to reflect about my Aunt Gene. As the disease progressed she no longer made sense, but it was wonderful to just sit and hold her hand and listen to her respond as I told her stories of the past. She always smiled and answered back. It did not matter to me that I could not understand her disjointed phrases. She was a supportive Aunt in my life and I felt good about visiting her. I thought of how she was there for me when my father died and always had kind words of encouragement. She attended my wedding and Mom's 80th birthday party among other family activities. She was a rock for me and all family members. It was an opportunity to give back to Aunt Gene. Dearest sweet Aunt Gene, may you dance with the angels and rest in peace. Thank you for being my aunt.

Chapter 11:

MARCH

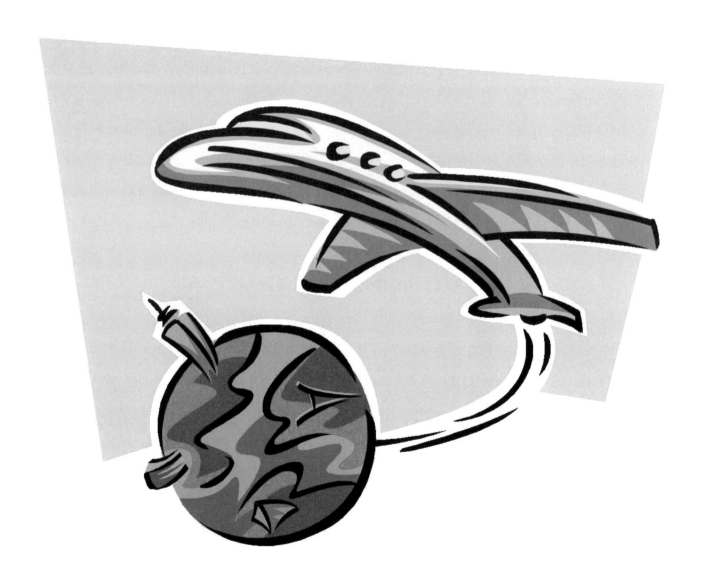

Happy St. Patrick's Day!

Making a Shamrock Sponge Painting

Good project for end of second-stage to middle of third-stage Alzheimer's.

Supplies needed:
6 sponges, each 2 $\frac{1}{2}$ x 3 inches (you can cut large sponges in half).
Green tempera paint.
Shamrocks cut from the pattern found on page 144.
Newspaper.
Masking tape.
2 small containers for paint.
Styrofoam plates.

Instructions: Cover a table big enough to seat 6 comfortably with sheets of newspaper, tacking it down with masking tape. Place several extra sheets of newspaper at each resident's working area to absorb the paint, as the residents will be painting beyond the outer edge of the shamrocks.

Place two containers of paint on the table. (Make sure you use a container that they won't associate with food! One time in the facility an activity assistant noted that a resident drank blue paint!) Place a styrofoam plate, a shamrock, and a sponge at each seat. Pour a little paint onto each plate. Bring in residents. Introduce project: "St. Patrick's Day is tomorrow and I thought it would be fun to decorate some shamrocks for your room." Demonstrate the project: Place one white shamrock on the newspaper. Dip the sponge in green paint on the plate. Sponge paint the shamrock (a little white will show).

The project is completed for their room!

Pattern for the Shamrock Project

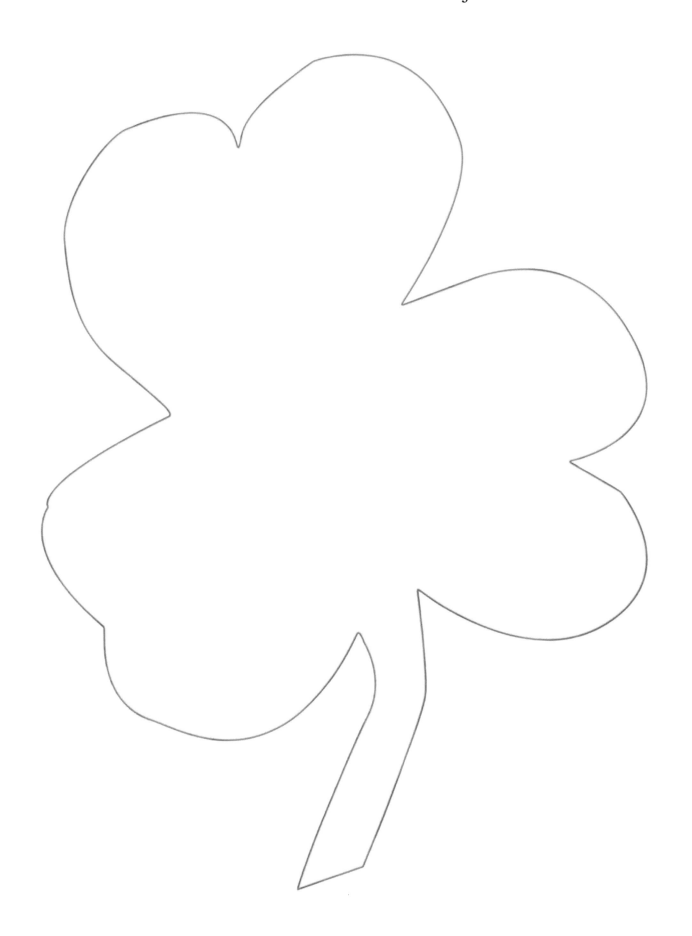

Completed Project

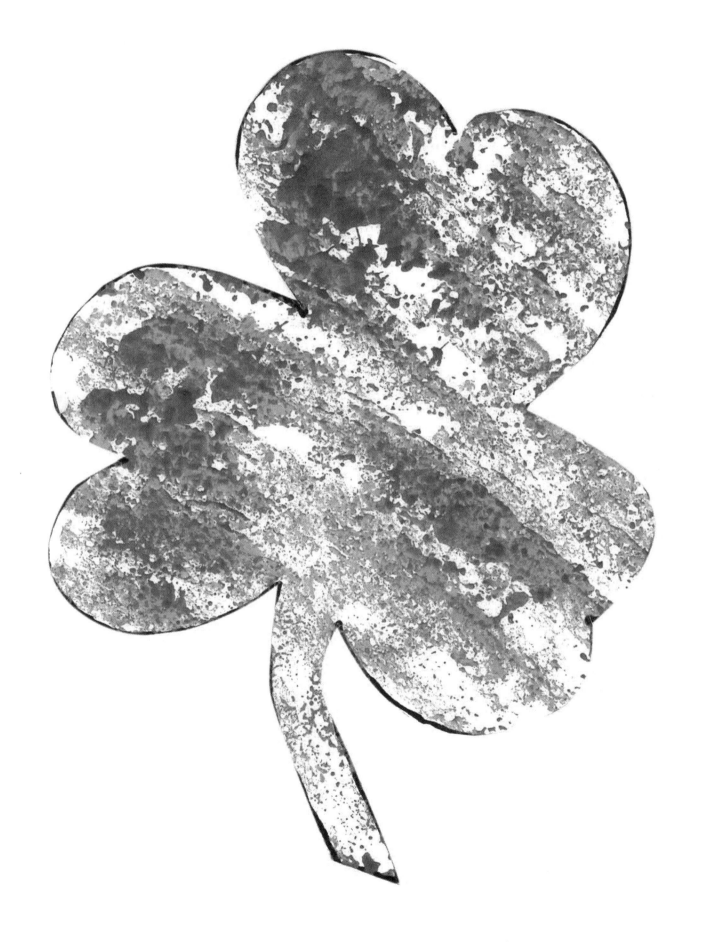

A Wee Bit of Irish St. Patrick's Day Party

I read Irish cards to the the residents and shared good Irish cheer. I asked what they used to do on St. Patrick's Day. Some could recall that they wore green in honor of St. Patrick's Day. I also dressed up in green and wore an Irish hat. I had a pot of "gold" and pictures of leprechauns and shamrocks. I played Irish songs on my accordion and sang with the residents.

"Danny Boy"

"Harrigan"

"I'll Take You Home Again, Kathleen"

"The Kelly Dance"

"Killarney"

"Kitty of Coleraine"

"A Little Bit of Heaven" (Sure They Call It Ireland)

"McNamara's Band"

"The Minstrel Boy"

"Mother Machree"

"My Wild Irish Rose"

"Rory O'Moore"

"The Rose of Tralee"

"Sweet Rosie O'Grady"

" 'Tis the Last Rose of Summer"

"Too-ra-loo-ra-loo-ra" (an Irish lullaby)

"The Wearing of the Green"

"When Irish Eyes Are Smiling"

"Where the River Shannon Flows"

"Who Threw the Overalls in Mistress Murphy's Chowder?"

"The Harp That Once Through Tara's Halls"

"Irish Washerwoman"

St. Patrick's Day Shamrock Cake

Yield: One 9x13-inch cake

Preheat the oven to 350 degrees. Following the directions on the box, prepare batter for a two-layer or 9 x 13-inch white cake. Add a few drops of green food coloring to the batter. Mix well, and pour into a 9 x 13-inch greased pan. Bake for 35-40 minutes. Frost with **Pistachio Frosting:**

Mix 1 box (3/4 ounce) pistachio flavored instant pudding mix and one pound frozen non-dairy whipped topping, thawed, and beat until smooth. Use half to frost cake. Using a shamrock cookie cutter, at random press several shamrock shapes on the frosted cake. Fill a pastry bag with the remaining frosting and outline the shamrocks. Refrigerate cake overnight.

St. Patrick's Day Punch

Yield: Three quarts
2 cans (1 quart each) pineapple juice
1 quart 7-Up
A few drops green food coloring
1 pint lime sherbet

In a large punch bowl, mix pineapple juice and 7-Up. Add the green food coloring and mix together. With an ice cream scoop, form balls of sherbet and float in the punch. Let the lime sherbet melt a bit into the punch and serve with the cake.

Hawaiian Theme Party

The purpose of the party is for stimulation, exercise, and fun. Get the staff to dress in Hawaiian clothing. Set the table with a Hawaiian theme, using a tablecloth patterned with pineapples, palm trees, or hibiscus flowers. Let the residents touch the cloth as you point to the various Hawaiian decorations. Place a length of fishnet in one area of the table and cover with colorful seashells. Add a floral centerpiece of silk Hawaiian-style flowers.

Place a lei around each person's neck and give each one a Hawaiian straw hat. Let the residents look at themselves in a mirror. Tell them that a lei shows love. Have name tags and a magic marker on hand. Look up each resident's name on the list on opposite page to find its Hawaiian counterpart, or let the resident pick a Hawaiian name they like. Write both their real and Hawaiian names on the name tag. Place the name tag on their shirt or blouse.

Cut into a fresh pineapple and let them smell it and touch the rough skin. Show a sugar cane stalk and let them touch it. If you can't get a sugar cane stalk, show a picture of one. Tell them that these two crops (sugar cane and pineapple) are the leading ones in Hawaii. Tell them that "aloha" means both "hello" and "goodbye." Have them say "aloha" with you. Play a Hawaiian music CD and wear a hula skirt.

Do the hula dance with the residents to work with their arms and hands. Place their arms above their heads in a circle to form a sun. Move their hands in a back and forth motion at chest level to imitate birds flying. Get fingers to move up and down touching the thumb as if Hawaiian people are talking. Only a few will be able to do these exercises. The residents with the end of third-stage to beginning of fourth-stage Alzheimer's can watch and enjoy the music and movements. If a staff member can sing and play a guitar or ukulele, the group can sing various Hawaiian songs. I've found that Hawaiian music is both soothing and upbeat, and the residents really light up when they hear it.

"Blue Hawaii"	"Aloha Oe"
"Tiny Bubbles"	"The Breeze and I"
"One More Aloha"	"The Hawaiian Love Call"
"Our Love and Aloha"	"The Moon of Manakoora"
"The Hawaiian Wedding Song"	"Now Is the Hour"
"I'll See you in Hawaii"	

Serve chilled Hawaiian punch at the party. (To prevent choking, do not put ice in the residents' glasses.)

Hawaiian Names

Alfred	Alapai	AH-luh-PAH-ee	Abigail	Apikalia	AH-pee-kuh-LEE-uh
Arthur	Aka	AH-kuh	Agnes	Akeneki	AH-keh-NEH-kee
Bernard	Pelenalako	PEH-leh-nuh-LAH-koh	Ann, Anne, Anna	Ana	AH-nuh
Bert, Burt	Peka	PEH-kuh	Beatrice	Peakalika	PEH-uh-kuh-LEE-kuh
Bill	Pila	PEE-luh	Bernice	Pelenike	PEH-leh-NEE-keh
Carl, Karl	Kala	KAH-luh	Bessie	Pakake	puh-PAH-keh
Charles	Kale	KAH-leh	Betty, Bette, Betsy	Peke	PEH-keh
David	Kawika	KAH-VEE-kuh	Charlotte	Halaki	hah-LAH-kee
Donald	Konala	koh-NAH-luh	Clara	Kalala	kuh-LAH-luh
Dwight	Kuaika	koo-AH-ee-kuh	Dolores	Kololeke	KOH-loh-LEH-keh
Earl, Earle	Ele	EH-leh	Dorothy	Koleka	KOH-LEH-kuh
Edgar	Ekeka	eh-KEH-kuh	Edith	Ekika	eh-KEE-kuh
Edward	Ekewaka	EH-keh-WAH-kuh	Edna	Ekena	eh-KEH-nuh
Elmer	Elema	eh-LEH-muh	Emma	Ema	EH-muh
Eugene	Iukini	EE-oo-KEE-nee	Eunice	Eunike	EH-oo-NEE-keh
Francis	Palakiko	PAH-luh-KEE-koh	Florence	Pololena	POH-loh-LEH-nuh
Fred	Peleke	peh-LEH-keh	Grace	Kaleki	kuh-LEH-kee
Gerald	Kelala	keh-LAH-luh	Helen	Helena	he-LEH-nuh
Harold	Halola	hah-LOH-luh	Irene	Ailina	AH-ee-LEE-nuh
Henry	Hanale	HAH-nuh-LAY	Jane, Jean, Jenny	Kini	KEE-nee
Howard	Haoa	HAH-oo-uh	Joan, Joanne	Io'ana	ee-OH'-AH-nuh
John, Jon	Keoni	keh-OH-nee	Katherine	Kakalina	KAH-kuh-LEE-nuh
Joseph	Iokepa	EE-oh-KEH-puh	Lily	Lilia	lee-LEE-uh
Lawrence	Lauleneke	LAH-oo-leh-NEH-keh	Louisa, Louise	Luika	loo-EE-kuh
Leonard	Leonaka	LEH-oh-NAH-kuh	Marcia	Malakia	MAH-luh-KEE-uh
Martin	Makini	mah-KEE-nee	Margaret	Makaleka	MAH-kuh-LEH-kuh
Norman	Nomana	NOH-MAH-nuh	Marie, Mary	Malia	muh-LEE-uh
Philip	Pilipo	pee-LEE-poh	Miriam	Miliama	MEE-lee-AH-muh
Ralph	Lalepa	lah-LEH-puh	Nell, Nellie	Nele	NEH-leh
Raymond	Leimana	LEH-ee-MAH-nuh	Patricia	Pakelekia	puh-KEH-leh-KEE-uh
Richard	Likeke	lee-KEH-keh	Pauline	Polina	poh-LEE-nuh
Robert	Lopaka	loh-PAH-kuh	Rebecca	Lepeka	leh-PEH-kuh
Ronald	Lonala	loh-NAH-lah	Ruth	Luka	LOO-kuh
Stanley	Kanale	KAH-nuh-LAY	Susan, Susannah	Kukana	koo-KAH-nuh
Steven, Stephen	Kiwini	kee-VEE-nee	Theresa, Teresa	Keleka	keh-LEH-kuh
Theodore, Ted	Keokulo	KEH-oh-KOH-loh	Victoria	Wikolia	vee-KOH-LEE-uh
Thomas, Tom	Koma	KOH-muh	Vivian	Wiwiana	VEE-vee-AH-nuh
Vernon	Wenona	veh-NOH-nuh	Yvonne	Iwone	ee-VOH-neh
Walter	Walaka	wah-LAH-kuh			
William	Wiliama	WEE-lee-AH-muh			

Chapter 12:

APRIL

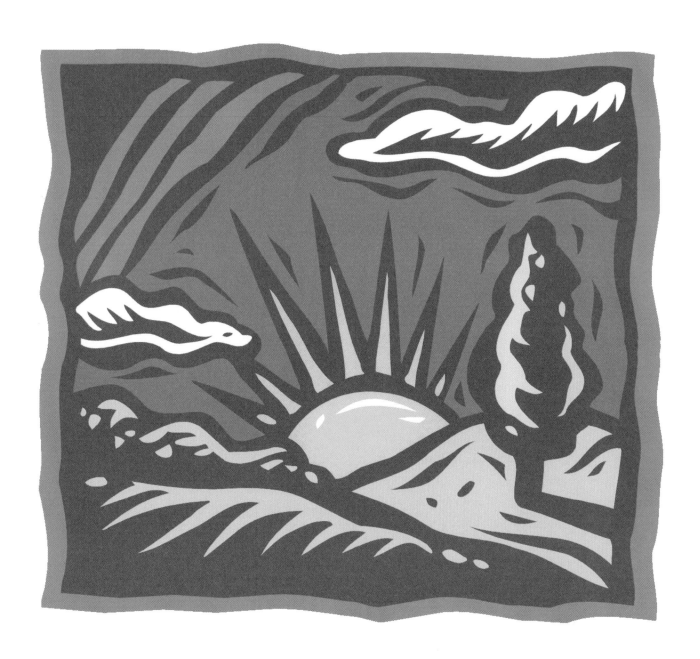

Signs of Spring Weather

Supplies needed:

> Big umbrella.
> Small parasol to block out the sun.
> Sunglasses.
> Rain jacket with hood.
> Rubbers.
> Hat with visor.
> Birdsong clock or bird guidebook.
> Outdoor thermometer.
> A range of spring flowers and plants such as daffodils, hyacinths, chives, mint, dandelions, pussy willows, pinecones, Brussels sprout stalk or head of cabbage, tree twigs with buds or blossoms. (Local farmers, gardeners, or grocery stores may be able to help you with these.)

I brought my big wooden clock that tells the temperature, the time, and the humidity. The residents loved this clock. A rough cedar birdhouse with a bright red cardinal painted on it was also a hit. I played a CD called "Thunder" with the sound of rain, birds singing, and the sound of storms. I handed out rhythmic instruments to the residents, such as bells, tambourines, a triangle, wooden sticks, and a small drum. Some of the residents enjoyed playing the instruments while others hummed along or just listened. One lady covered her ears with her hands and said please make the thunder go away. A couple told about their fear of thunder as a child. One resident said whenever it thundered she climbed under the bed and hid until the thunder stopped. Another lady said that her dad held her in his arms when it thundered and talked about the storm until she calmed down. Some talked about the puddles of water they waded through after the storm. It was fun to hear them reminisce.

I carry a large doll with me named Lucy Mae who has pantaloons, tattered suede shoes, big pigtails, a cotton dress and hat to match. I held her and talked to them about her playing in the rain and mud. Her pigtails were wet. They felt the wet pigtails. We talked about drying her pigtails and making sure she was dry.

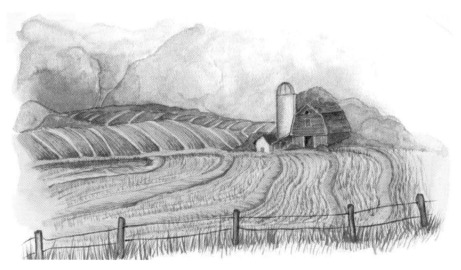

Create a Story Picture

This picture is used to help residents recall tornadoes on a farm or an area where they grew up. It could be a good picture for a topic on the weather.

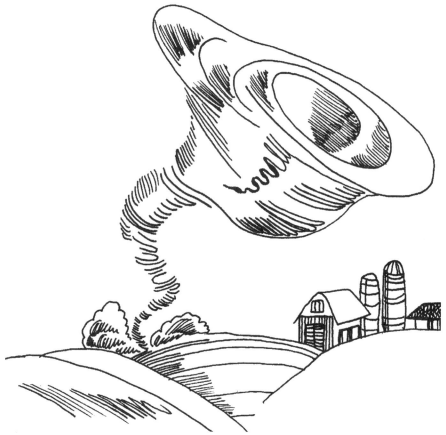

You can run off copies. Ask the residents what they see in the picture. This is a good exercise for First-and Second-stage Alzheimer's patients. They can also color in the picture.

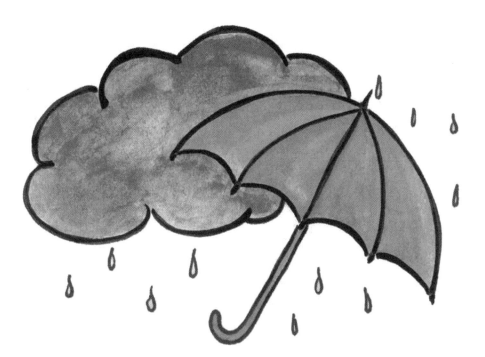

Next, I showed off the clothes that are worn when it rains and opened the large umbrella. I asked them if they are superstitious about opening an umbrella indoors. Then I let them see how the umbrella will shield them to keep them dry and showed off the fancy parasol that shields them from the sun. When I did this, they liked the bright colors on the umbrella. I put on the sunglasses to show how their eyes are also protected from the sun. Let them touch the clothing and umbrellas to feel the texture. Talk to them about rain that drizzles. Let them listen to the rain on the CD.

Next the birds will start singing. Point out the robin in the guidebook. It surprised me that one lady identified the robin's picture. She loved birds and always had birdhouses and bird feeders while she was living in her home. Another woman identified the cardinal on the cedar birdhouse. The men in the group also enjoyed feeling the roughness of the wood on the birdhouse. We talked about the robin as being a sign of spring.

Use a picture of a tornado as a conversational piece. One man mentioned that lightning had struck his barn and also talked about a tornado in his area. The picture helps to generate memories and conversation.

I walked around the room with a bunch of spring flowers so the residents could smell the sweet fragrance. I loved to watch each person's face as they were smelling the flowers. The residents rubbed mint leaves on their hands and smelled the clean fragrance. They also enjoyed the smell of fresh chives. I brought in a stalk of Brussels sprouts that was still in the ground from last year's harvest. The odor was very pungent. The reactions on the faces were very interesting to watch. They definitely could tell the difference between the pungent smell of a Brussels sprout stalk and the sweet fragrance of a spring flower.

In between the show and tell, conversation, and scents, I played songs on my accordion about the weather. You can play tapes instead or just sing with them. As I played the music and sang with them, I enjoyed watching them tap a foot or wiggle their body to the music.

A list of songs to jog memories related to words about spring weather:
"Home on the Range" (Not cloudy all day)
"On a Clear Day" (clear)
"He's Got the Whole World in His Hands" (wind and rain)
"Whispering Hope" (sunshine)
"Amazing Grace" (sun)
"I Found a Million Dollar Baby" (April shower, rain)
"The Birth of the Blues" (breeze)
"Emilia Polka" (rainy weather)
"Rain, Rain" polka (rain)
"I Love Paris" (spring)
"April in Paris" (spring)
"You'd Be So Nice to Come Home To" (breeze)
"Spring Will Be a Little Late This Year"
"The Last Time I Saw Paris" (spring)
"May The Good Lord Bless and Keep You" (sunlight, rain)
"The Rain in Spain" (rain)
"Wrap Your Troubles in Dreams" (cloudy and gray)
"You Are My Sunshine" (sun)
"Lazy River" (sun, shade)
"I'm Looking Over a Four-Leaf Clover" (rain)

Rainbows

I started my program by playing and singing "Somewhere over the Rainbow." Next I showed pictures of rainbows in various outdoor scenes. I asked how many had seen a rainbow. Then I asked questions: What do you like about the rainbow? When does a rainbow appear? Wouldn't it be exciting to be able to grab hold of a rainbow? Do you know how a rainbow is formed? It is made possible by the sunlight shining through the water molecules in the air. Do you realize that the sun is a big star? It is over ninety million miles away from the earth. The sun is a huge ball of gas with temperatures of 6,000 degrees.

Usually you see a rainbow in arc form. However, if you were flying in an airplane, the rainbow would appear like a circle. The airplane would fly right through the center of the rainbow. On the ground you need to turn your back to the sun in order to see the arc of the rainbow. You can find rainbows in a fine spray of a fountain, waterfall, or after a rainstorm. You can take a hose and spray a mist of water in the sunlight to form a rainbow too. The best time to see a rainbow is right after a rainstorm early in the morning or late in the afternoon. If the light is blocked you will only be able to see part of the rainbow. There are primary rainbows. What colors could you see in this rainbow? Red is at the top and violet is at the bottom. Orange comes after red, then yellow, green, blue, and violet. Sometimes you can see a rainbow in reverse. Then the red would be at the bottom of the rainbow and violet at the top. If you were going to make the color orange you would have to blend together red and yellow. To make green mix yellow and blue.

We baked a 9x13-inch cake. I made a batch of frosting and we mixed the colors of the rainbow and filled cake tubes with the different colors. We worked with the residents to make a primary rainbow on the cake. We had cake and coffee. The residents really enjoyed the activity. We concluded with the song "When You Wish Upon a Star" in honor of the sun.

"Each of us has a unique capacity to help discover the colors in our very own rainbow." —Author unknown

Use this rainbow to show the residents the colors in a rainbow.

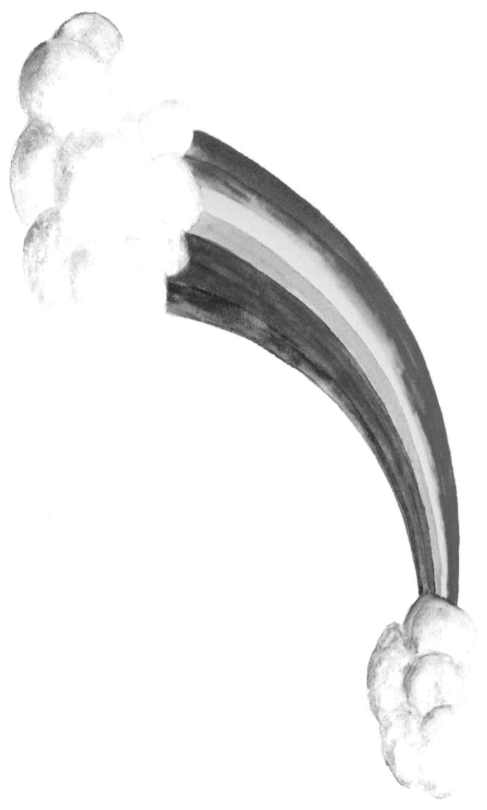

The Magic of an Egg

Invite a local chef from a restaurant or culinary arts student to come in and put on a demonstration on how to make an omelet. The person dressed like a chef has a great impact on the residents. A staff member may do the job instead.

Omelet:

Yield: 15 small pieces for tasting

- 1 tablespoon margarine
- 1 tablespoon chopped shallot or onion
- 2 tablespoons diced ham
- 1 tablespoon diced green pepper
- 1 tablespoon milk
    Salt and pepper to taste
- 4 eggs, beaten

Melt margarine in omelet pan over medium heat. Sauté shallots, ham, and green pepper for 2 minutes. Add milk, salt, and pepper to the beaten eggs. Pour over the sautéed meat and vegetables. Loosen sides as the omelet begins to coagulate. When omelet is firm and loosened from the bottom of the pan, flip omelet over in air and catch it in the pan. Those who are not on a restricted diet may have a taste of the omelet.

The purpose of the demonstration is watching the order the dish is put together, noting the smell as it cooks, tasting the omelet, skill of cracking an egg.

Eggs: A Sensory Stimulation Exercise

Supplies needed:

Small eggs
Medium eggs
Large eggs
Jumbo eggs

Put the small egg against the large egg and jumbo egg, and the medium against the small egg and large egg to compare sizes. Residents can crack an egg of each size into a bowl. Inspect the size of the egg yolks. Afterward, let a resident beat the eggs. Cook scrambled eggs.

Show the residents a brown egg. The brown egg jogs memories. One person said, "We used to get a lot of brown eggs on our farm." Ask them if they've ever smelled a rotten egg. My dad used to say, "Boy, that person is a rotten egg."

Songs to Go With the Theme:

"I'm Putting All My Eggs in One Basket"

(Words and music by Irving Berlin)

I'm putting all my eggs in one basket,

I'm betting everything I've got on you.

I'm giving all my love to one baby

Lord help me if my baby don't come through.

I've got a great big amount saved up in my love account honey

and I've decided love divided in two won't do.

So I'm putting all my eggs in one basket.

I'm betting everything I've got on you.

Read the words to the residents, then play and sing the song.

The Chicken Song

"The Chicken Song" is a polka. This song has no lyrics.

Get the staff or volunteers to do the chicken dance with the residents as the music plays. Teach the residents to put hands under their armpits and move their elbows up and down to form flapping wings. Teach them to clap and get the staff to turn around in a big circle. The residents can sit in wheelchairs and use their arms and hands for exercise. They enjoy the beat to this song.

She'll Be Coming 'Round the Mountain

Verses:

> She'll be coming 'round the mountain when she comes,
>
> She'll be carrying Grannie's brown eggs when she comes,
>
> Oh we'll all go out to meet her when she comes,
>
> She'll be wearing eggs on her hat when she comes,
>
> Oh we'll all have eggs and bacon when she comes,
>
> Oh we'll all sing about eggs when she comes.

I got an old straw hat and hot-glued plastic eggs on it. You can purchase plastic eggs in a craft store. I also carried a small basket of brown eggs. I recommend wearing a hat and bib overalls to play the part. It creates a lot of conversation and fun as you model your outfit.

Chapter 13:

MAY

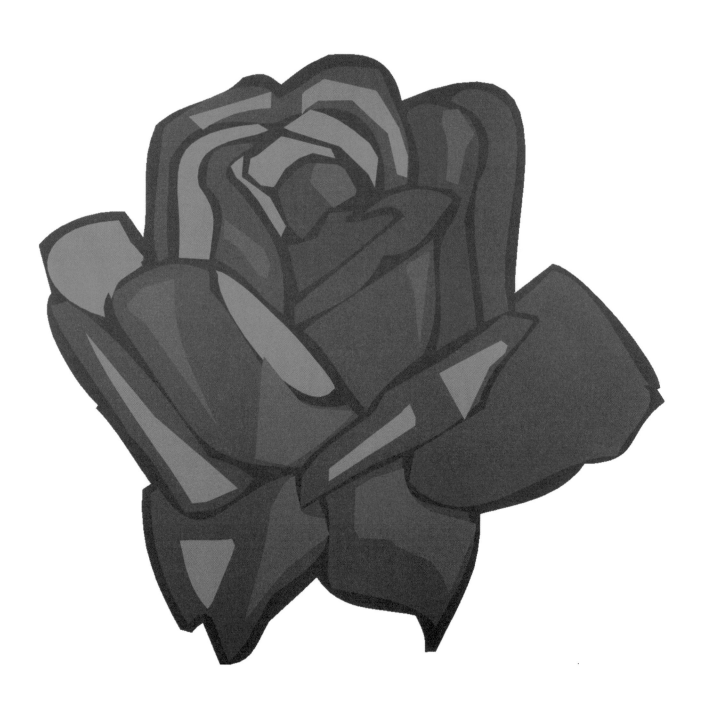

Stringing Cheerios

Supplies needed:
> Yarn.
> Tape.
> Cheerios, or other donut-shaped cereal.
> Scissors.

Cut yarn into desired lengths. Wrap tape around one end of each piece of yarn to form a "needle" (this looks like a shoelace). Give each resident a length of yarn. Slide the first Cheerio down to the end of the yarn and tie a knot to secure it. The residents seem to enjoy this craft and like the idea that the finished strings will be used to feed the birds and animals outside. The exercise is good for their hands and fingers. Also it is okay for the residents to eat the Cheerios. One lady ate as many Cheerios as she strung on the yarn. We were lucky to have families donate yarn and Cheerios.

It is a great project that allows people to interact with each other. We had a little ceremony putting the finished strings on the trees outside to feed the birds, and the folks enjoyed the nice weather in late May.

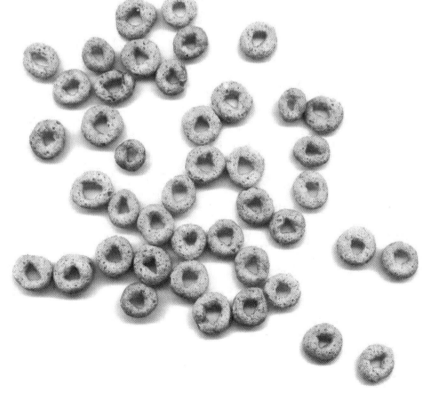

Mother's Day Project: A Mini Fashion Show

Match colors and put together items to make an outfit.

Part I: Shoes

Supplies needed:

6 pairs of shoes in different styles.

6 shoe boxes.

Scramble six pairs of shoes in the middle of the table. Get the residents to pair up the shoes and place them into the shoe boxes. Make sure you have different colored shoes with different textures. Let the residents feel the textures of the shoes and describe them. Ask, "Is this shoe soft, or smooth, or rough?"

Part II: Outfits

Supplies needed:

6 women's outfits.

6 pairs of shoes, one to match each outfit.

6 purses, one to match each outfit.

6 hats, one to match each outfit.

Show one outfit and two pairs of shoes. Ask which pair of shoes goes with the outfit. Show two hats and then two purses with one outfit and ask which hat and purse matches best with the outfit.

Once the selection has been made, put the shoes, purse, and hat all together for the residents to see.

Let the residents feel the hats, purses, and dresses or suits. Place the hats on the residents and lay the suit up against the resident's body. Let the resident look in the mirror to see how they look.

The residents enjoyed this exercise thoroughly. One husband came to see his wife while we were doing this exercise. He sat in on the activity and watched. After the activity was completed he said that his wife really loved shoes. She had a pair of shoes for every outfit and every occasion. He said she kept taking his side of the closet with all of her shoes. He finally built three extra shelves to the ceiling of the closet to take care of the problem. She filled those shelves and still used his side of the closet. He said to me, "You like pretty shoes too—I bet your husband has to fight for closet space too."

"No," I said. "He finally got smart and got his own closet."

I had a silver dress and silver shoes that matched, but I also had a pair of black shoes with silver lining. One resident said that the black shoes with the silver lining go with the silver dress. I had not thought of it like that before. She was matching the silver dress with the silver lining in the shoes. I said, "Sure enough, that definitely goes with the silver dress."

I concluded the program with the following poem:

MOTHER

M   is for the million things she gave me.

O   only means she is growing older.

T   is for the tears she shed to save me.

H   is for the heart of gold.

E   is for everything she gave me and

R   is for right and right she always will be.

   Put them all together and they spell mother, a word that means a world to me.

Making Cards

Supplies needed:

Wallpaper sample books (your local decorating place will donate old wallpaper books to your care center).

Scissors.
White 8$\frac{1}{2}$ x 11-inch copy paper.
Glue stick.
Pens (1 per resident).
Rulers (1 per resident).

The purpose of the project is to get the residents to pick out the piece of wallpaper they like to make a card. This exercise helps the resident make choices and also express their feelings, likes, and dislikes. This exercise makes the resident happy. Making choices makes the resident feel he/she is in control.

Note: *If at all possible, get a couple of volunteers involved in this project, as well as a second activity person.*

Give each resident one wallpaper book. Help the resident page through the book. Let each resident talk about color and shape preferences. Once they pick out a pattern, they like to rip out the wallpaper page.

Fold the wallpaper in half. Use a ruler to make the size of card desired. Cut on the line. Cut the $8^1/_2$ x 11-inch copy paper the same size as the wallpaper. Glue the white paper to the inside of the card. Ask the resident what she would like to say and write it in for her. Many third-stage Alzheimer's patients have forgotten how to write. After I helped a resident to make up a card of her choice, she was all smiles and proud of the card. When I asked her what would you like the card to say. She said, "Peaches gives thanks!"

Another woman was in the end of the second-stage of Alzheimer's and could no longer write. She had done a lot of artwork all of her life, and she made a card with little help. She wanted to send it to her son and daughter-in-law. I asked her what she wanted to say. She said, "Tell them I am thinking of my dear son and daughter-in-law. I hope you have a beautiful day. I love you, Mom." I was amazed at her thoughts. I wrote inside the card for her and sent it to the family. Two weeks later I received a long-distance call from her son. He was very moved by the card. He had not received a card from his mom in years. It is a wonderful feeling to be touched by deep emotion.

That's Amorè Pasta Party

In 1968 I traveled to Europe while working on my master's degree. One of the countries I visited was Italy. I was amazed at the architecture and the culture. I took a snapshot of Venice with people in a gondola. My cousin used colored pencils and made a large sketch of the scene for me. I had it framed and have enjoyed the picture greatly. There are four people in the gondola. One man is using an oar to move the boat along in the water while the other three people are just riding along. Two other boats are in the scene, along with a clock tower. Many buildings are near the dock nearby. I took my treasure into the care facility to share with the residents. You can do this project with any picture of Italy.

I told them that they were going to create a story. I began by asking if anyone knew which city in Italy this was. One man said it was Venice. "You are right," I exclaimed. I asked the residents what they would like to call the story. They decided on "Venice." I had a volunteer student document the story. Each resident could tell what they saw in the picture as I asked questions about the picture.

"Where do you think these folks are going today?" I asked.

Mae said, "They are going to war and getting there by riding the boat." Lois thought they were just taking a ride and having fun in the water. Elizabeth said, "They are going sightseeing." Ann said, "They are going to church and then they will have a party." Hank said, "I know where I would go if I were in that boat. I would be going fishing and catch those big ones. Then I would pan-fry all the fish. It would be fun." Ralph said he would be going to see the Venetian buildings.

Other questions: What kind of weather do you think it is in this picture? There is another boat with two people; where do you think they are going?

The above is just an example of how to create a story with a picture of a foreign place. You can use this technique for 30 to 60 minutes or as long or short as you like. The residents get the opportunity to express themselves. There are no right or wrong answers. The residents had fun and enjoyed the creative activity. Do not put words into their mouths or make up their story. Let them say what they want to say.

I brought in an Italian flag and a colorful map of Italy. I pointed out some of the major cities in Italy: Rome, Venice, Naples. They enjoyed the flag and the map. One man recalled traveling to Italy in his younger days and really looked over the map when I passed it around.

> I then played Italian music:
> "Addio, Addio" (goodbye)
> "Arrivederci Roma" (goodbye to Rome)
> "Ciribiribin" (Chiribiribee)
> "Come Back to Sorrento" (Torna A Surriento)
> "Cosi Cosa"
> "Farewell Dear Napoli"
> "Funiculi, Funicula" (a happy heart)
> "La Dolce Vita" (the sweet life)
> "My Hearts Belongs to You" (Amore Un'Altra)
> "O Sole Mio" (My Sun)
> "Oh Marie" (Maria, Mari!)
> "Rome Will Never Leave You"
> "Serenade"
> "That's Amorè" (That's Love)
> "Three Coins in the Fountain"
> "Volarè"
> "You Don't Have to Say You Love Me"

I encouraged the residents to identify and feel the texture of a variety of dry pastas I had brought in: spaghetti, seashells, manicotti, macaroni, wagon wheels, and rigatoni. They all recognized and named the spaghetti and seashells.

I passed out linguine which is flat and spaghetti that is rounded (the pasta was not cooked). Some of the residents twirled the piece of spaghetti between their thumb and forefinger. They then tried to twirl the linguine and some said, "Oh, it's flat." One resident said she had made lots of spaghetti as a high school cook. The kids used to come and see her. They would have contests to see who could take a string of cooked spaghetti and suck it into their mouths. She said they were fun to watch as they had a good time.

I passed around the following spices and talked about them and their uses in cooking as they smelled them: gourmet garlic seasoning, Italian seasoning, onion powder, pizza seasoning, pasta seasoning, crushed fresh garlic, garlic paste, parsley, and fresh onion.

I melted butter in a pan and sautéed one diced onion and one minced clove garlic. I added 1/2 pound of cooked spaghetti, pizza seasoning, onion powder and Parmesan cheese to taste. They enjoyed the smell of the pasta. I concluded the program with "Yankee Doodle Dandy" because the song has the word "macaroni" in it. I sang the song with them. We also sang, "Hey Good Lookin', What You Got Cookin'?" The residents enjoyed the spices, conversation, and music.

Chapter 14:

JUNE

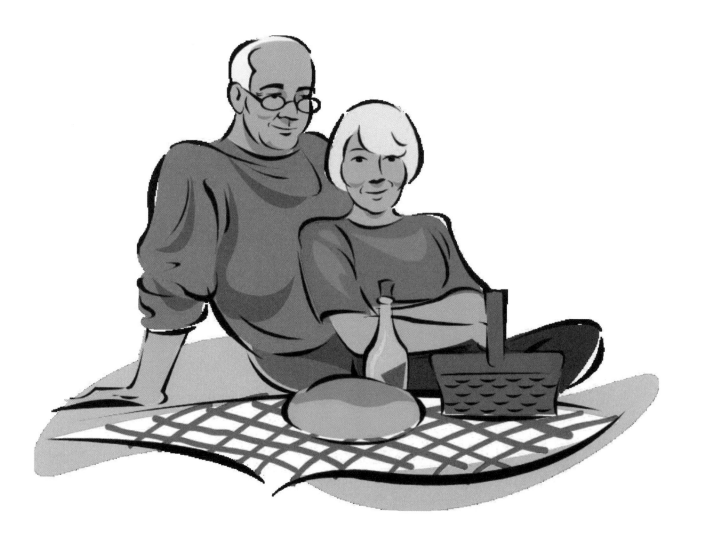

Hugs Program

I traveled to various nursing care facilities with the Hugs program. It was well received by the residents and staff. Basically it is a sing-along that adds a little spice to each resident's life. The program runs 45 minutes to an hour.

I give every resident a coupon at the beginning of the program (see below). It is good for one free hug and can be redeemed whenever needed. You can use teddy bears, hearts, clowns or other symbols on your coupons. It will warm your heart to see sad faces turn to smiling faces.

I read the following:

"A hug is all natural. It is naturally sweet, has no preservatives, no artificial ingredients, and is 100 percent wholesome. A hug is almost perfect. You need not purchase batteries like for the Energizer Bunny because it gives an automatic high energy yield. It is tax free. There

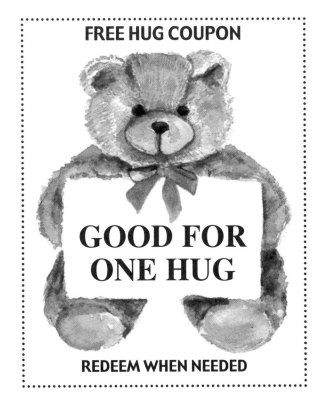

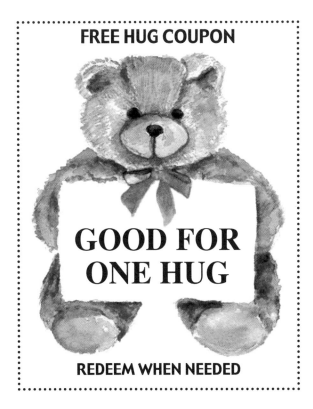

are no monthly payments, no insurance requirements, and no prescriptions for medicine. It is fireproof, theft-proof, non-polluting. It is fat-free and inflation-proof. The best part is that it is fully refundable. It lowers blood pressure and cholesterol, and regulates the heartbeat. Hugs add to an individual's emotional, mental, and physical well-being. It is good therapy due to user-friendly physical contact. It strengthens the immune system. Hugging a hyperactive child can be calming to the child. You need at least four hugs to survive the day. It is suggested that eight hugs is best for maintenance and twelve for growth."

When the program is over ask to get a hug. Most of the residents will hug you. I played music related to the theme:

> "I Love You Truly"
> "Ave Maria"
> "When I Fall in Love"
> "Love Is in the Air"
> "Let Me Call You Sweetheart"
> "True Love"
> "Why Do I Love You?"
> "Easy to Love"
> "Anniversary Song"
> "How Deep Is Your Love"
> "Let's Fall in Love"
> "All The Things You Are"
> "Could I Have This Dance?"
> "When the Saints Go Marching In"

When I play the song "When the Saints Go Marching In," I would get the residents to march their feet in place pretending they are marching for hugs. Then add a hand motion—even a snapping of fingers. Not every resident will be able to snap their fingers. The idea is to have the residents exercise their bodies to the best of their ability and have fun. Exercise the eyes by getting the resident to blink their eyes. See if the residents can wink one eye at a time. Get the residents to smile. Get the residents to open their eyes wide and put on a happy face. Play the song "Put On a Happy Face." Next get the residents to frown. These are great exercises

HUGS

It's wondrous what a hug can do,
A hug can cheer you when you're blue.
A hug can say, "I love you so."
Or, "Gee! I hate to see you go."

A hug is, "Welcome back again!"
And, "Great to see you!" or "Where've you been?"
A hug can soothe a small child's pain
And bring a rainbow after rain.

The hug! There's just no doubt about it,
We scarcely could survive without it.
A hug delights and warms and charms,
It must be why God gave us arms.

Hugs are great for fathers and mothers,
Sweet for sisters, swell for brothers,
And chances are some favorite aunts
Love them more than potted plants.

Kittens crave them. Puppies love them.
Heads of state are not above them.
A hug can break a language barrier,
And make the dullest day seem merrier.

No need to fret about the store of 'em.
The more you give, the more there are of 'em.
So stretch those arms without delay
And give someone a hug today.

—Author unknown

for the facial muscles. I always point out that it takes more muscles to frown than to smile.

Sing songs about eyes ("Beautiful Brown Eyes," "When Irish Eyes are Smiling"). Check out the folks that have brown eyes versus blue, green, or gray eyes. Count up the number of residents with each eye color. Talk to each resident about the color of their eyes.

My mother had beautiful blue eyes. She loved to hear the caregivers tell her she had the most beautiful blue eyes. In fact she would cooperate with the caregivers after they complimented her about her eyes.

Play and sing "Kumbaya"

Verses:
> Someone's hugging, Lord, Kumbaya…
> Oh, Lord, Kumbaya.
> Someone's kissing, Lord, Kumbaya…
> Oh, Lord, Kumbaya.
> Someone's smiling, Lord, Kumbaya…
> Oh, Lord, Kumbaya.
> Someone's loving, Lord, Kumbaya…
> Oh, Lord, Kumbaya.
> Someone's singing, Lord, Kumbaya…
> Oh, Lord, Kumbaya.

Conclude the program with "Let Me Call You Sweetheart."

Flag Day, June 14

At the turn of the last century, a schoolteacher named Bernard Cigrand hung the American flag out the door of the schoolhouse. In 1916 he persuaded President Woodrow Wilson and Congress to declare Flag Day a national holiday. Flag Day is celebrated on June 14. Many cities host Flag Day parades. Appleton, Wisconsin, holds the largest parade in the country in honor of the American flag. The first Flag Day was celebrated at Stony Hill School on June 14, 1887, near Waubeka, Wisconsin (just north of Milwaukee).

Raise the flag and salute it, saying the "Pledge of Allegiance".

One-on-one Visit

Daughter and mother with a flag activity.

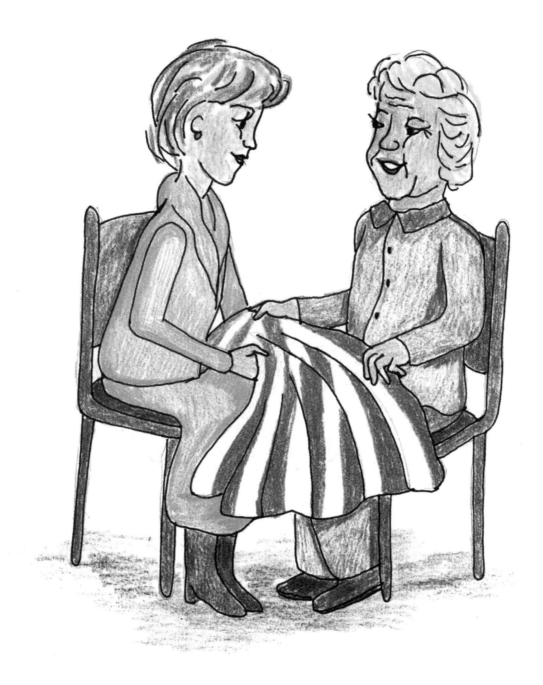

Play the following songs and clap with the music.

"Stars and Stripes Forever"

"American Patrol"

"Washington Post"

"Our Director March"

Hand out American flags and get the residents to wave the flags with the music.

Play and sing the following patriotic songs.

"It's a Grand Old Flag"

"America"

"Yankee Doodle"

"This Is my Country"

"God Bless America"

"Star Spangled Banner"

"Marine Hymn"

"When Johnny Comes Marching Home Again"

"Battle Hymn of the Republic"

"Dixie"

"Caissons Song"

"The Battle Cry of Freedom"

"America the Beautiful"

"This Land Is My Land, This Land Is Your Land"

"Yellow Rose of Texas"

"Home on the Range"

Recite or read the poem "My Land Is Fair for Any Eyes to See," (p. 229, *Favorite Poems Old and New*, by Helen Ferris). Conclude by playing and singing "Amazing Grace."

Father's Day Lunch

I set up in a special room. I put tablecloths on the table and made nature-themed center-pieces. The kitchen brought down meals to the men. We served nonalcoholic beer and sparkling grape juice.

I invited a guest speaker to talk to the men about what it was like to be a Dad. Many were mentally alert and some were in early stages of Alzheimer's or had some form of dementia. They enjoyed reminiscing about their lives and their children. The speaker did an excellent job leading the various topics and getting the men involved in the conversation. They enjoyed the extra attention and the fact that they could be with all men.

Note: Dementia is the Latin word for "out of mind".

Summer Cookout

The purpose of the program is awareness of the season. Stimulate the senses with barbecue and picnic spices, and have residents recall what they would do on a summer day, using a picture to prompt memories. They also will have fun and relax.

The picture I use is full of greenery and flowers by a mill and farm. There are flowers everywhere and lush grass. The barn is not far away. It is a beautiful sunny summer day. The cool breeze is gently blowing. There is trout pond nearby. It is a perfect day for a barbecue.

Present the picture and ask the residents what they would do if they were in this picture. Some of the responses were as follows: I would lay down in the green grass and just enjoy the hot sun. I would pack some food and visit with my family. I would plant flowers by the barn. I would fish by the pond. I would enjoy the weather. I would walk around and take in the sights. I would have a party.

As I studied their backgrounds, it is interesting to see that the person who wanted to plant was a gardener and the person who wanted to fish had enjoyed fishing as a hobby. The person who would enjoy the hot sun had traveled in the tropics. The person wanting a party had had many parties and entertained. These are just a few examples. This exercise gives people an opportunity to reflect.

We talked about the fresh air, and the birds, and nature. A lady said, "Nature is so beautiful and has so much to offer us." I presented two pictures with one bird in each picture, sitting in a birch tree. One gentleman could identify the cardinal and another lady identified the blue jay. I then presented the group with the bark of the birch tree. They enjoyed seeing and touching the bark.

Seasonings used:
Chili powder.
Liquid smoke.
Garlic pepper.
Spicy salsa seasoning.
Southwestern seasoning.
Smoky seasoning.
Barbecue seasoning.
Smoky mesquite seasoning.
Gourmet garlic seasoning with salt.
Premium blend table spice .
Salsa seasoning.

We passed the seasonings around and let the residents smell the spices as we imagined the great smells of the air and the good smells of a barbecue cooking. We talked about making Mexican chicken with chili powder, barbecued ribs with liquid smoke, smoky seasoning on beef and turkey.

Southwestern seasoning was great for making baked beans. Garlic pepper would add extra flavor to corn on the cob. Smoky mesquite marinade was great on beef. Gourmet garlic seasoning would be great for roasting a pig.

One lady said, "You are making me hungry talking and thinking of all this food!" We then made Quick 'n Easy Salsa.

Quick 'n Easy Salsa

1   can (14^1/$_2$ ounces) tomatoes with diced green chilies

1   tablespoon salsa spice (dehydrated green peppers and onions)

Place tomatoes into a frying pan. Add the salsa spice. Cook until salsa comes to a slow boil. Stir and simmer for 3-5 minutes. Cool.

Note: *The residents enjoy the smell of the salsa. I did not serve the salsa to them because it is spicy hot.*

I then played the following songs for the residents:

"Oh What a Beautiful Morning"
"Beautiful Dreamer"
"Wouldn't it Be Lovely"
"Those Lazy Hazy Days of Summer"
"Summertime"
"You Are My Sunshine"
"In My Merry Oldsmobile"
"Down By the Old Mill Stream"
"Sweet Adeline"
"On the Street Where You Live"
"Ain't We Got Fun"
"I'm Looking Over a Four-Leaf Clover"

Some of the residents tap along or move their arms. Some hum the tunes. They enjoy the music. We concluded the program with the song "Till We Meet Again."

Chapter 15:

JULY

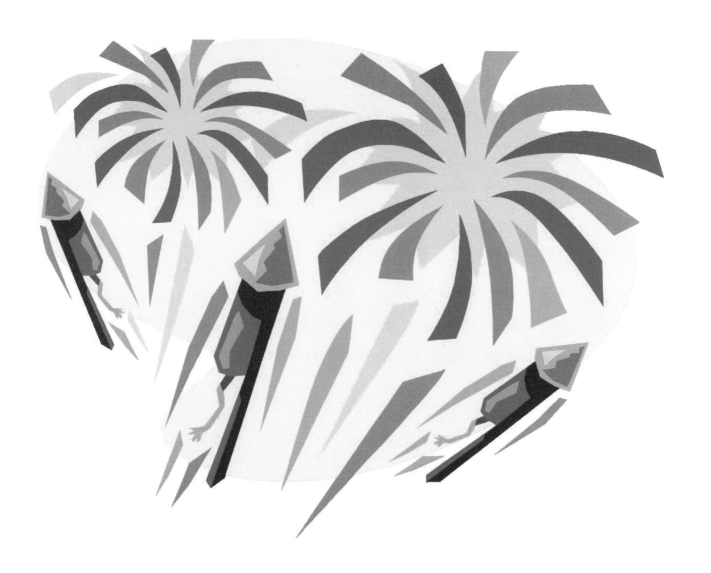

Betsy Ross

Betsy Ross was born in Philadelphia, Pennsylvania, on New Year's Day, 1752. She was named Elizabeth Griscom, and her family called her Betsy. Her mother and father were Samuel and Rebecca. She was the eighth child of seventeen children. The Ross family were Quakers, who lived in a peaceful manner. Because the family was so large, everyone had to do chores. Betsy was assigned to make the white caps that Quaker girls were required to wear every day. Betsy went to Friends School with other Quaker children. She learned the three R's in addition to geography. For her daily service project each day after school, she sewed quilts and samplers. She won many prizes for her beautiful needlework.

Betsy wanted to work outside her parents' home in her later teenage years. They consented to have her work for an upholsterer. There she met and fell in love with John Ross. She married John against her parents' wishes—he wasn't a Quaker. John and Betsy set up a shop called Ross Upholsterer. They worked together long and hard hours.

At the time, America was made up of thirteen colonies under the ruler King George III of England. In 1775 the Continental Congress put together an army to fight the British. The Revolutionary War began in Lexington and Concord in Massachusetts. The Philadelphians knew about the war but it did not interfere with business in their city.

Betsy's husband joined the army and later was injured in an explosion. Betsy tried to nurse John back to health, but he didn't recover. Betsy then ran the shop alone. After work she made musket balls, a job that was at odds with the peace-loving Quakers' beliefs.

General George Washington wanted an American flag made. John's uncle suggested that Betsy Ross make the flag. George Washington sketched a design. Colonel Ross, Robert Morris, and George Washington met at Betsy's shop in Philadelphia to discuss the making of the flag. This flag had 13 stripes (seven red and six white) and 13 stars to symbolize the colonies.

They sat by the fire with the teakettle heating water for the men while discussing the making of what would later be known as the Betsy Ross Flag.

Betsy studied the design very carefully and said, "A five-pointed star would be easier to make. A six-pointed star like in your design would waste material. I don't really like a square flag, sir. I think a rectangular flag is the classic style." George Washington was impressed by Betsy's observation and agreed to let her embellish on his suggested design. Betsy took great pride in making thirteen white five-pointed stars on a blue field. She stitched the blue field against the red and white stripes.

The Declaration of Independence was signed on July 4, 1776. On June 14, 1777, the minutes of the meeting read:

"Resolved that the flag of the United States be thirteen stripes alternating red and white, that the union be thirteen stars in a blue field representing a new constellation."

Due to her excellent work on the flag she gained much respect and her upholstery business grew. She was a hardworking woman and well respected. This was very unusual for a time when women had very little power, yet she managed to run a business from her home and raise a family.

Betsy married a second time, to Joseph Ashburn. He died in an English prison. She then married a third time to John Clypoole. Betsy raised five children and outlived three husbands. She taught sewing to her nieces, daughters, and grandchildren. Betsy retired at the age of 75 due to failing eyesight. She was quite a storyteller. Her favorite story was about the making of her flag. It was her grandson William Canby that made Betsy Ross' story public. She died at the age of 84 in 1836. She was buried in Arch Street in the garden of her upholstery shop. The United States flag flies over her grave 24 hours a day.

Suggest to the residents that they salute Betsy Ross on this July 4 for her outstanding work on the first American Flag in the spirit of 1776 by playing and singing "It's a Grand Old Flag."

Pass out Betsy Ross flags and have the residents wave the flags with the song.

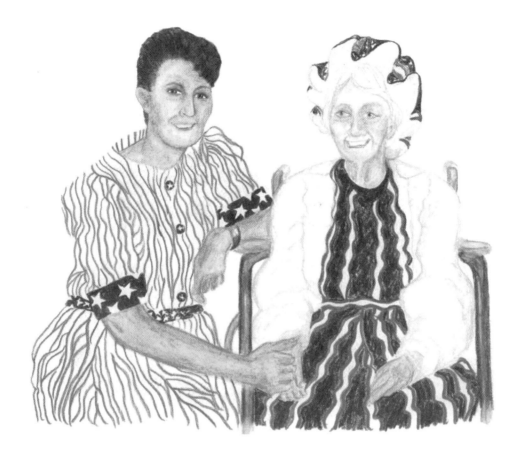

One of the songs that I sang with the residents was "Kumbaya." I changed the words and called it "The Flag Song." (Throughout this book I used the "Kumbaya" melody and change the words to fit the program. It is a very familiar song to the residents. The repeated melody is simple for Alzheimer's residents to follow.)

"The Flag Song"

Wave the flag my friends, Kumbaya.
Oh, Lord, Kumbaya.
Salute the flag my friends, Kumbaya
Oh, Lord, Kumbaya.
Raise the flag my friends, Kumbaya
Oh, Lord, Kumbaya.
Hail the flag my friends, Kumbaya
Oh, Lord, Kumbaya.
Honor the flag my friends, Kumbaya.
Oh, Lord, Kumbaya.

I dressed up like Betsy Ross to tell the story. I also dressed up a resident with a revolutionary hat and apron. I set up a scene where George Washington, Colonel Ross, and Robert Morris met for tea in Betsy's home. I had a teakettle boiling and made tea to let the smell permeate the room. I got the residents to repeat after me about the story of Betsy Ross and the making of the flag. I have material of the flag that residents can feel and see. We talk about the parts of the Betsy Ross flag and their meanings. We took pictures of the resident "actors" and "actresses." The residents had fun. Conclude the remaining program with other patriotic songs.

> "My Country 'Tis of Thee"
> "Stars and Stripes Forever"
> "God Bless America"
> "American Patrol"
> "Yankee Doodle Dandy"
> "This Land Is Your Land"
> "Marine's Hymn"
> "Battle Hymn of the Republic"
> "Dixie"
> "This Is My Country"

The marches, such as "American Patrol" and "Stars and Stripes Forever," are good numbers to have the residents clap or tap along to. If they can no longer clap they can shake a rhythmic instrument, alone or with a little help. Take time to talk about the meaning of the words in each song.

I ended the program by repeating the song "You're a Grand Old Flag."

Celebrating Our State

Since I live in Wisconsin, I researched facts about our state and shared them with the residents. There is a great sense of pride in Wisconsin. People are hard workers and have a strong sense of family. There is a sense of loyalty to parents, and many people care for their elderly parents at home.

You can do this project with any state, with a bit of simple research. I have a big flag of

Wisconsin that I lay out on a table for the residents to inspect. The flag shows the state's emblems and tells its history. I also have a map of the state which we spread out and use to spark conversation about places in the state the residents are familiar with. We discuss all the things associated with Wisconsin, and I have them guess what the answer is for each item.

Flower:	Wood violet.
Tree:	Sugar maple.
Wild animal:	White-tailed deer.
Insect:	Honeybee.
Mineral:	Galena.
Fish:	Muskellunge or muskie.
Soil:	Antigo silt loam.
Rock:	Red granite.
Animal:	Badger.
Bird:	Robin.
Domestic animal:	Holstein Friesian cow
	(Each year the cow of the year is a different breed).
Song:	"On Wisconsin".
Fossil:	Trilobite.
Dog:	American water spaniel.
Beverage:	Milk.
Grain:	Corn.
Dance:	Polka.

I then play a variety of polkas. Then I put on some recorded polka music and I go around and dance with the people in their wheelchairs, clapping hands and exercising their arms. It is good stimulation for each person.

Dancing is a good activity for other reasons as well. Many elderly people went dancing at ballrooms in their younger days and some even met their mates at the ballrooms. This brings back so many beautiful memories for them. One of the songs that Wisconsin residents like is "In Heaven There Is No Beer." The residents usually guess that the beverage in Wisconsin is beer. For some of the parties we serve nonalcoholic beer, particularly for the men's group. We also show off the University of Wisconsin's sports teams' Badger flag and sing "On Wisconsin." One of the men mentioned there is nothing like a cold beer while watching a football game.

I bring in samples and/or pictures of the following:

Violet.

Sugar maple leaf and some bark.

White-tailed deer.

Honeybee. You can bake some biscuits and put butter on the biscuit. Use a honey dipper to drizzle the honey on the biscuit. The
smell of the biscuits baking will help keep some of sleepy residents awake. Some of the residents can butter the hot biscuits
and help drizzle the honey over them. I like to watch their faces
while they help do this task. There are many happy faces as they
anticipate eating the warm biscuits.

Galena.

Muskie.

Red granite.

Holstein Cow.

Song (I bring in the music and words to "On Wisconsin" and recite
and sing the words).

American water spaniel.

Milk. I always have a glass of milk available, and I ask the residents
why we drink milk. One said to have healthy bones. Another
resident said he liked milk with his cookies.

Two ears of corn. I let the residents feel the silk and husks and ker-
nels of one of the ears. I cook the ear of corn that has not been
passed around, and they can smell the aroma of the fresh corn
cooking. I melt butter and have the residents brush the butter
over the corn.

For this activity it isn't necessary to have samples and pictures of every item. You can
select a few and have a conversation with the residents. Choose the items that you feel the residents are most familiar with and interested in to help you get residents involved in the project.

For example, the men in the group really enjoyed the muskie and the badger. A lot of the
men had fished in their day. One gentleman had a stuffed muskie hanging in his room. So I
borrowed it for conversation about celebrating our state.

Emblems of Our State

Much of Wisconsin's story is told on the state flag and other state symbols. The flag was designed many years ago when mining and shipping were important industries in Wisconsin. Our flag shows a sailor and a miner holding a shield between them. The shield is divided into four parts. These parts show a plow (for farming), a pick and shovel (for mining), an arm holding a hammer (for manufacturing), and an anchor (for shipping).

Below the shield is a horn of plenty filled with fruits and other foods, which represent Wisconsin's crops. The bars of lead to the right of the horn are for Wisconsin's rich minerals. At the top is the state motto, "Forward," above our state animal, the badger. (On some versions of the flag there is an arc of thirteen stars under the horn of plenty, representing the country's first thirteen states.)

Flags

The purpose of this exercise is to feel the material; to recognize shapes, sizes and colors; to stimulate the mind and to provide enjoyment of the various flags. The elderly are very patriotic and appreciate the meaning of flags.

Supplies needed: A variety of pictures of flags from various countries. I bring in the actual flags whenever I can; pictures of all the flags listed below are on the following pages.

Chinese flag	German flag
Mexican flag	Libyan flag
Italian flag	Malaysian flag
Canadian flag	Cuban flag
Japanese flag	Puerto Rican flag
Rwandan flag	Polish flag
Greek flag	Irish flag
Lebanese flag	U.S. map in color

Some flags have birds, stars, etc. It helps residents to recognize the shapes and colors.

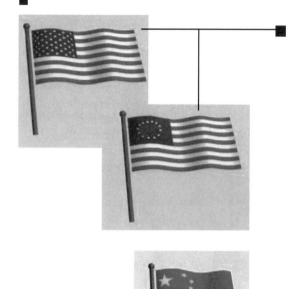

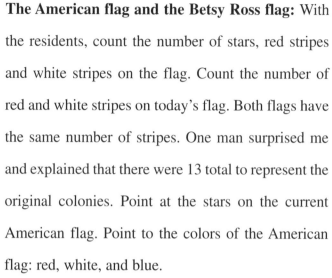

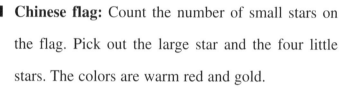

■ **The American flag and the Betsy Ross flag:** With the residents, count the number of stars, red stripes and white stripes on the flag. Count the number of red and white stripes on today's flag. Both flags have the same number of stripes. One man surprised me and explained that there were 13 total to represent the original colonies. Point at the stars on the current American flag. Point to the colors of the American flag: red, white, and blue.

■ **Chinese flag:** Count the number of small stars on the flag. Pick out the large star and the four little stars. The colors are warm red and gold.

■ **Mexican and Italian flags:** The flag colors of these countries are the same—green, red and white. Lay the flags side by side. Have the residents point to the snake, cactus, eagle, and wheat on the Mexican flag.

■ **Canadian flag:** Point to the object in the center of the flag. What shape is this object? What kind of leaf? What color is the maple leaf? Show an actual maple leaf if you live in an area where you can bring one in. The residents could touch the leaf and see the veins in the leaf.

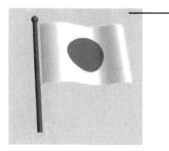

■ **Japanese flag:** Point to and touch the circle in the flag. Use a resident's finger to outline the shape of the circle on the flag to get a feel for the shape.

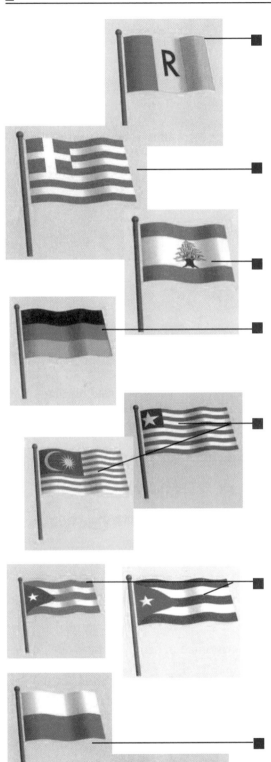

■ **Rwandan flag:** The flag is red, gold and green. See if the group can recognize the letter on the middle of the flag (R). Run the finger down the letter R to get a feel of the shape.

■ **Grecian flag:** The flag is light blue and white. Count how many blue stripes (five) and white stripes (four). Run your finger down the white cross.

■ **Lebanese flag:** The flag is red and white. Find and touch the tree on the flag.

■ **German flag:** Ask the residents how many colors are in the flag? Three: black, deep yellow and red. Touch each color as the color is named.

■ **Liberian and Malaysian flags:** Lay the flags side by side. Pick out the similarities. The Liberia flag and Malaysian flag both have stripes but the Liberian flag has only one star on the field while the Malaysian flag has the sun and moon on the field.

■ **Cuban and Puerto Rican flags:** Lay the flags side by side. The Cuban flag has a red triangle with a white star, three blue stripes and two white stripes, whereas the Puerto Rican flag has three red stripes and two white stripes with a blue triangle and a white star.

■ **Polish flag:** Note that this flag is red at the bottom and white at the top.

■ **Irish flag:** It has three vertical bands of color: green, white and orange.

You can use flags to stimulate conversation with the residents about their heritage. In Wisconsin, there are many Germans, Italians, Scandinavians, Irish, Poles, and people from Spanish-speaking countries. Sometimes a resident will want to see the flag of the country they are from. These activities help build a bond between activity director and resident and make it easier to work with residents.

The United States

I brought in a large colorful map of the United States made out of fabric. Each state has a picture with the name of the capital, bird, and flower.

I work with a small group of 6-8 people. We view the birds and flowers in some of the states that the residents select. I get the map out and talk about a few states at a time. Then I play patriotic music and our state song, "On Wisconsin." This is a very familiar song to Wisconsin residents. I also play "When the Red, Red, Robin Comes Bobbin' Along," since the robin is our state bird.

I once worked with a particular resident who could not remember her name. She had graduated from Yale and could sing that school song in perfect tune, word-for-word, but couldn't remember her name or recognize her family members, nor her own image. Another woman came from France and could sing the national anthem of France but could not recognize the national anthem of the United States, where she had lived for 70 years. Her family informed me she was a very patriotic person. Another gentleman played the harmonica in his younger days and was very interested in U.S. history. He carried his harmonica in his lap as he wheeled around the facility. One time I said, "Adolf, let's play and sing 'Oh Susanna' in honor of the state of Alabama." I began to play the tune on my accordion. He picked up the harmonica and played every note with me. His family was coming down the hall to visit him. Tears streamed down his son's and daughter-in-law's faces. He had not played the harmonica in years. We all applauded for him. I hugged him and thanked him for a job well done. Three days later he died in his sleep.

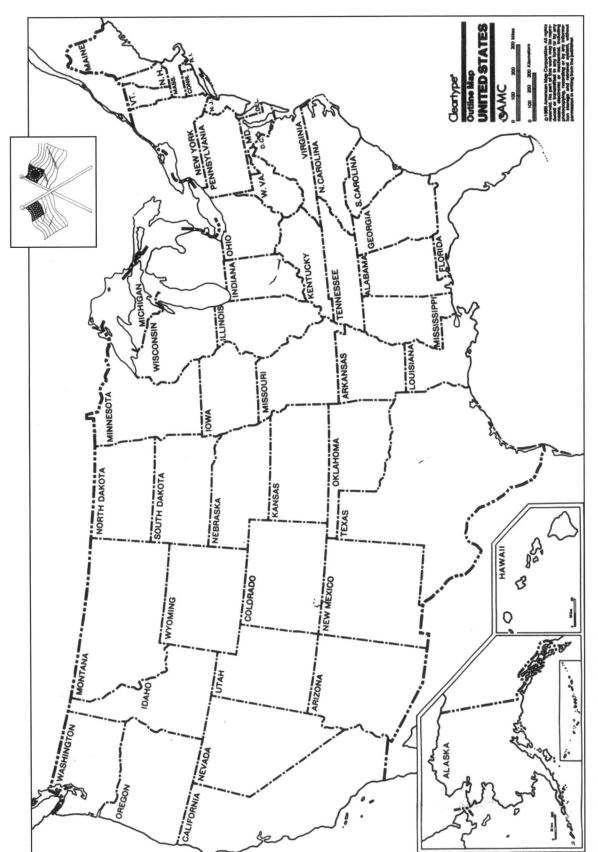

Note: Residents can color in the States.

My point is simple. You just don't know what, how, or when an Alzheimer's patient will respond as their mind is triggered by a memory. That is why caregivers and people who work with Alzheimer's residents must live for the moment.

I am a firm believer in the philosophy of love, laughter, and living for the moment. Rejoice when the Alzheimer's resident accomplishes the smallest task. Laugh with the residents and make life light and merry whenever possible. Love them no matter the situation for they are not the people they once were. Understand and meet their needs to the best of your ability. Remember to use your kindness and heart to help them get through their day. Above all, it is the little things that count for the Alzheimer's patients. Enjoy the new person they are when and wherever possible. Understand that they live in their own little world.

I asked questions of the residents: Where would you like to go to visit someone special? (They may not know the state but often they express a desire to visit a son or a daughter who lives far away.) What are some special memories you have from taking a trip? Did you take family trips? Do you remember where? (Some can recall the past while others cannot.)

Sizes of the States

They looked on my map for the three largest states, the smallest state and two states that a lot of people move and retire to. You can point out the states that surround the state that the residents live in. **Note:** *In some cases it's best to only pick one state from each of the above categories. Work within the limitations and abilities of the residents. Talk about the weather in various parts of the country. Weather is a familiar topic to discuss for most people as well as a good conversation starter.*

Play a few of songs containing the names of the states, such as "The Yellow Rose of Texas," "Arkansas Traveler," "California Here I Come," "Oh Susanna," "The Sidewalks of New York," "Sweet Georgia Brown," "Pennsylvania Polka," "Oklahoma," "On Wisconsin," "Mississippi Mud," "Blue Hawaii," "The Hawaiian Wedding Song," "My Old Kentucky Home,"

"Gary, Indiana," and "Back Home in Indiana," "Shenandoah." Locate these states one at a time and play the songs in honor of each state. Some residents will not be able to locate them. It does not matter. A gentleman who had earned his living as a history teacher could locate many of the states on the map while doing this exercise.

A List of States With Each Capital, Flower, and Bird

Alabama
Capital: Montgomery, flower: camellia, bird: yellowhammer

Alaska
Capital: Juneau, flower: forget-me-not, bird: willow ptarmigan

Arizona
Capital: Phoenix, flower: Saguaro cactus blossom, bird: cactus wren

Arkansas
Capital: Little Rock, flower: apple blossom, bird: mockingbird

California
Capital: Sacramento, flower: golden poppy, bird: California valley quail

Colorado
Capital: Denver, flower: blue columbine, bird: lark bunting

Connecticut
Capital: Hartford, flower: mountain laurel, bird: American robin

Delaware
Capital: Dover, flower: peach blossom, bird: blue hen chicken

Florida
Capital: Tallahassee, flower: orange blossom, bird: mockingbird

Georgia
Capital: Atlanta, flower: Cherokee rose, bird: brown thrasher

Hawaii
Capital: Honolulu, flower: hibiscus, bird: nene

Idaho
Capital: Boise, flower: mock orange, bird: mountain bluebird

Illinois
Capital: Springfield, flower: violet, bird: cardinal

Indiana
Capital: Indianapolis, flower: peony, bird: cardinal

Iowa
Capital: Des Moines, flower: wild rose, bird: American goldfinch

Kansas
Capital: Topeka, flower: native sunflower, bird: western meadowlark

Kentucky
Capital: Frankfort, flower: goldenrod, bird: cardinal

Louisiana
Capital: Baton Rouge, flower: southern magnolia, bird: brown pelican

Maine
Capital: Augusta, Flower: white pine cone and tassel, bird: black-capped chickadee

Maryland
Capital: Annapolis, flower: black-eyed Susan, bird: Baltimore oriole

Massachusetts
Capital: Boston, flower: mayflower, bird: black-capped chickadee

Michigan
Capital: Lansing, flower: apple blossom, bird: American robin

Minnesota
Capital: St. Paul, flower: showy lady's slipper, bird: common loon

Mississippi
Capital: Jackson, flower: southern magnolia, bird: mockingbird

Missouri
Capital: Jefferson City, flower: hawthorn, bird: eastern bluebird

Montana
Capital: Helena, flower: bitterroot, bird: western meadowlark

Nebraska
Capital: Lincoln, flower: goldenrod, bird: western meadowlark

Nevada
Capital: Carson City, flower: sagebrush, bird: mountain bluebird

New Hampshire
Capital: Concord, flower: purple lilac, bird: purple finch

New Jersey
Capital: Trenton, flower: violet, bird: American goldfinch

New Mexico
Capital: Santa Fe, flower: yucca, bird: greater roadrunner

New York
Capital: Albany, flower: rose, bird: eastern bluebird

North Carolina
Capital: Raleigh, flower: flowering dogwood, bird: cardinal
North Dakota
Capital: Bismarck, flower: wild prairie rose, bird: western meadowlark
Ohio
Capital: Columbus, flower: carnation, bird: cardinal
Oklahoma
Capital: Oklahoma City, flower: mistletoe, bird: scissor-tailed flycatcher
Oregon
Capital: Salem, Flower: Oregon grape, bird: western meadowlark
Pennsylvania
Capital: Harrisburg, flower: mountain laurel, bird: ruffed grouse
Rhode Island
Capital: Providence, flower: violet, bird: Rhode Island red
South Carolina
Capital: Columbia, flower: yellow jessamine, bird: Carolina wren
South Dakota
Capital: Pierre, flower: pasque flower, bird: red-necked pheasant
Tennessee
Capital: Nashville, flower: iris, bird: mockingbird
Texas
Capital: Austin, flower: Texas bluebonnet, bird: mockingbird
Utah
Capital: Salt Lake City, flower: sego lily, bird: California gull
Vermont
Capital: Montpelier, flower: red clover, bird: hermit thrush
Virginia
Capital: Richmond, flower: flowering dogwood, bird: cardinal
Washington
Capital: Olympia, flower: West Coast rhododendron, bird: American goldfinch
West Virginia
Capital: Charleston, flower: rosebay rhododendron, bird: cardinal
Wisconsin
Capital: Madison, flower: wood violet, bird: American robin
Wyoming
Capital: Cheyenne, flower: Indian paintbrush, bird: western meadowlark

Note: *The library has books with pictures of the flowers and birds of each State. You can put together your own booklet for the residents and also use this booklet as a one-on-one tool.*

Barbecue Outing

In the courtyard area, the staff grilled bratwurst and hamburgers. The kitchen prepared potato salad, baked beans, fruit, dessert, and beverages. We set tables up outside in the area and served the residents. It's a good idea to pipe in some music.

Set up a buffet table with the food using a summer beach scene or western theme. Push the residents' wheelchairs through the line so that they can see the buffet setup. Fix a plate for each the resident, allowing each to choose what they want to eat. (A person on a pureed diet or tube feeding should not be invited to eat this food. A woman whose mother ate pureed food would feed her mom and bring her down to listen to the music and enjoy the fresh air. Her mom, a former music teacher, enjoyed this very much.)

Potatoes

The potato is a very familiar and favorite food. I began my program by asking the residents if anyone knew how potatoes were grown. A couple of farmers in the group had grown potatoes and talked about the backbreaking job of digging them.

I brought in potatoes of various sizes. The residents picked out the largest potato immediately and expressed surprise about the size. One lady said, "That is a lot of potato to eat!"

I then asked the residents what kinds of potatoes they liked. One resident said, "I like mashed potatoes and gravy." What are some other kinds of potato dishes? Potato salad. A lady said she always used up her Easter eggs in potato salad after Easter. "Fried potatoes are very good at breakfast", someone said, "scalloped potatoes and baked potatoes."

Fried potatoes

Supplies needed:

Potatoes.

Canola oil.

A range of seasonings, such as:.

Roasted potato seasoning mix.

Seasoning mix for spaghetti sauce.

Taco seasoning.

Chili seasoning.

Teriyaki seasoning.

Barbecue seasoning.

Mesquite seasoning.

I told them that we were going to do fried potatoes with various kinds of seasoning. First, we are going to see and smell some unusual seasonings.

I passed the seasoning around to the residents and named each seasoning. They enjoyed the good smells. Next I made fried potatoes with each seasoning.

Slice the potatoes, leaving them unpeeled. Heat 3 tablespoons canola oil in a skillet. Add one type of seasoning to a small batch of potatoes. Add potatoes to the hot oil. Fry a seasoned potato slices at a time until fork tender. Drain on a paper towel. Repeat with remaining potatoes and seasonings, one seasoning at a time. Pass the potatoes around for sampling.

Chapter 16:

AUGUST

Music and Aroma Therapy

Supplies needed:

A variety of potpourri fragrance candle chips of different scents. I used the following: rose, peach, apple, cinnamon, vanilla, spice, cherry, strawberry, lavender, and floral.

I left the scented candle chips right in their boxes. I passed the boxes around the table for each person to smell. They enjoyed the good smells. After each fragrance I played songs about the scents.

It seems that most residents like the smell of roses. They really liked it when I brought in roses from my garden in August. In fact, I brought in my last tea rose of the summer from my garden.

A lady in the group really smelled the rose scent. It is wonderful, she said. "My son grows roses in his garden. He brings in his roses just for me." I asked what colors does he grow. She replied, "He grows pink and red. Beautiful!" Does he grow tea roses? "No! He grows the big ones, you know! Just think, my baby son grows roses. I never knew he had it in him to grow roses."

Rose songs:

"My Wild Irish Rose"
"Roses Are Red"
"One Dozen Roses"
"The Last Rose of the Summer"
"Rose Leaf Rag"
"The Yellow Rose of Texas"
"When You Wore a Tulip" (and I wore a big red rose)
"San Antonio Rose"
"The Rose of Tralee"

Peach songs:

"Peach Picking Time in Georgia"
"Peach Time Rag"
"Peaches and Cream"

Apple songs:

"Don't Sit Under the Apple Tree"

"Apple Blossom Wedding"

"Apple Sass Rag"

"Apple Strudel"

"Apples and Bananas"

"Apples, Peaches, Pumpkin Pie"

"Ida"

"In the Shade of the Old Apple Tree"

Cinnamon songs:

"Cinnamon and Clove"

"Cinnamon Girl"

"Cinnamon Street"

Vanilla songs:

"Vanilla Ice Cream"

"Ice Cream"

Spice songs:

"Spice Up Your Life"

Cherry songs:

"Cherry Pink and Apple Blossom White"

"I Gave My Love a Cherry"

"Cherry Pies Ought to Be You"

"Cherry Oh Baby"

"Life Is Just a Bowl of Cherries"

Strawberry songs:

"Today"

"Strawberries Forever"

"Strawberry Wine"

Lavender song:

"Lavender's Blue"

Floral songs:

"Daisy" (Bicycle Built for Two)

"Edelweiss" (blossoms)

The program should be 30 to 50 minutes long depending on the amount of time devoted to music therapy. The residents play rhythmic instruments and some will hum or sing with the music while others are contented just to listen. Encourage participation and relaxation.

Grandma's Kitchen Activity

Follow the recipe for Mom's Old-Fashioned Beef Stew on page 135. Peel potatoes, carrots, and onions. Clean celery. Cut up the vegetables. Also, make a batch of muffins to go with the stew, and ask the kitchen staff to prepare jello salad, brownies, and beverages.

Set up the activity area with tables. Place tablecloths or placemats and a centerpiece on each table. Have the residents help you put out the place settings. Decorate the room to make it look special. Hire entertainment to come in for after dinner to sing to the residents. They really enjoy this type of program immensely.

This is a project you can do once a month using different theme foods.

Soda Can Vase

Supplies needed (for each vase):

1	soda can.
1	sheet tissue paper.
27"	length of ribbon.
1	fresh or silk flower.
1	fern.

Take off the ring at the top of the soda can, and fill it half full with water before decorating, if you're using fresh flowers. Make sure the can is dry before continuing.

Cut a 13-inch square from a sheet of tissue paper in colors to match your theme. (Each sheet will yield two squares.) Wrap the piece of tissue paper around the can. Tie the ribbon around the can. Tie a bow and curl the tails of the ribbon. Place a flower and fern in each soda can.

This centerpiece is very inexpensive to make, and it is easy for the residents to get involved in this simple project.

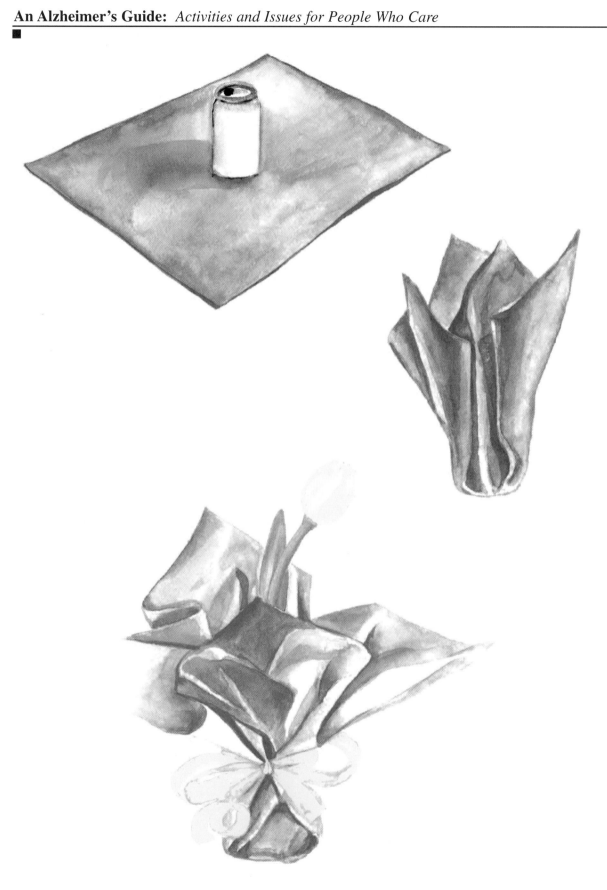

You can use fabric and ribbon to do the same project. You can also use newspaper to wrap the can. Comic strips are colorful and fun, and you can read them while making the vase!

We used these vases for the gathering at Grandma's kitchen. A sticker was placed underneath one place setting at each table. That resident won the flower centerpiece for his/her room. The winners were delighted with their prizes.

Camping Trip Party

Tell this story to set the scene:

Just before school started, I went camping with my family. Blacky, our cocker spaniel, came along too.

We packed a couple of tents, camping equipment, and of course food and eating utensils. Sometimes the evenings were a bit nippy so everyone packed an extra long sleeved flannel shirt and warm jacket to take the chill off of our bones. Dad built a campfire, and we sat around the fire and sang folk songs.

The smells of pancakes, bacon, and scrambled eggs in the early morning hours at the campground were mouth-watering. Our family often took a hike before breakfast. We all helped make breakfast and clean up the dishes. Blacky swam in the lake and came back to the campsite all wet with his fur covered with sand. He sat and waited for the pancakes. Often Blacky begged food from our family. The whole family fussed over that old dog. Blacky always had plenty of leftover pancakes. Now our family goes camping each year just before school starts again. What a memory!

Supplies needed:
Tent.
Sleeping bag.
Air mattress with pump.
Camping stove.
Old-style camping coffeepot.
Rhythm instruments, including bells, tambourine, cymbals.

Suggested campfire folk songs:

"I've Been Working on the Railroad"

"Oh Susanna"

"Oh My Darling Clementine"

"She'll Be Coming 'Round the Mountain"

"Michael Row the Boat Ashore"

"Red River Valley"

"Shenandoah"

"Home on the Range"

"Get Along Little Dogies"

"Frankie and Johnnie"

"Down in the Valley"

"Bury Me Not on the Lone Prairie"

"Jimmy Crack Corn"

"Nine Hundred Miles Away"

"Skip to My Lou"

"Deep River" (has the word campground)

(Country music)

Reference *The Giant Book of American Folk Songs* by Hal Leonard. It is a book of songs celebrating America's heritage.

Set up the tent. Let them feel the different fabrics of the tent and the sleeping bag. I have bright red plaid flannel in my sleeping bag. They can see and feel the air being pumped into the air mattress.

Corn Muffin Pancakes

Yield: 8-10 pancakes

2 tablespoons oil

1 egg

$3/4$ cup 2 percent or skim milk

1 small box ($8 1/2$ ounces) corn muffin mix

Heat griddle over camping stove or grill. Add oil, egg, and milk to the corn muffin mix in a bowl. Blend until the batter is just moistened. (Some participants can help stir the pancake mix by hand.) Pan is hot enough when a few drops of water sprinkled on the pan dance on the surface. Pour about 1/4 cup batter on hot griddle for each pancake. Turn pancakes when bubbles form and edges begin to dry.

Pancake Syrup

Yield: 1 cup

       2 cups brown sugar
       2 cups water
       2 teaspoons vanilla

Combine brown sugar and water. Heat on the camping stove until syrup comes to a boil. Add vanilla just before serving.

Walk around the group and help the participants crack a total of 4 eggs into a bowl and beat the eggs with a wire whisk. Scramble the eggs when the pancakes are done. Brew a pot of coffee to get the aroma in the area. Pass around the food to let them enjoy the smells. The residents with no diet restrictions can sample the eggs and pancakes. The good smells in the room and the participation make for some happy faces. Next, play music pretending we are around a campfire. Let the residents clap and/or play rhythmic instruments.

I play songs on my accordion. I talk about each song. Activity staff help the residents play the instruments and clap. Some will hum or move their body as the music plays.

Once while flipping a pancake I broke one pancake apart. I said, "This one will be for Blacky." A resident said, "My dog Blacky never went camping with the family. He stayed home and was in my backyard most of the time."

Another resident after the program squeezed my hand and said, "This was something a little different. I enjoyed it very much." Dare to be different!

On a sunny day this activity can take place outside.

The Farm Story

The purpose of this story is to try to jog the resident's memories while walking them through the four seasons of the year. A couple of the residents vividly remember how to milk a cow. Some talked about being very cold during the snowy winter days. A couple of the men remembered fishing.

After telling the residents the following story, we made chicken and dumplings with their help. This brought back a lot of memories. My own grandma made chicken and dumplings for her family every Sunday. She killed the chickens in her backyard. I still can vividly see the chickens hanging from the post. Once I watched a chicken running down the street without its head attached. It is a weird feeling to see this happen. My mom would say that she felt like a chicken running around without her head when she would get stressed out with too many things to organize and accomplish for the day.

Tell the Residents This Story:

Mom and Dad grow up together on neighboring farms. They married in 1909. Mary was their firstborn child in 1910. Dad was disappointed for he wanted a son. Five years later Mom was expecting for a second time. Dad made it very clear that Mom had better have a boy. Dad was shocked at the new arrivals. They were twin boys. Dad named his sons Daniel and Donald after his twin uncles. Twins ran in the family on Dad's side. Our family called the boys Dan and Don.

Dad and Mom were nervous about having twins at first. Dan was a happy baby, but Don was colicky. He was fussy and high-strung. He sometimes would keep the family up most of the night. Morning came awfully early.

There were always plenty of chores to do seven days a week. Milking cows was only one of the daily chores.This job was very time-consuming. After working long hours Dad sometimes complained of the soreness in his arms because he worked so hard plowing the land.

Mom used to rub his arms with her own homemade oil to help him feel better.

Sometimes Dad and Mary rode the tractor together. He never let Mary drive the tractor because he felt she was too young. Mary and her dad enjoyed their rides together. It gave Mary time to be with her dad.

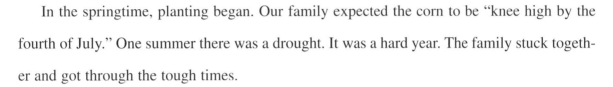

In the springtime, planting began. Our family expected the corn to be "knee high by the fourth of July." One summer there was a drought. It was a hard year. The family stuck together and got through the tough times.

Dad believed a man has to take care of his finances and pay the bills. Food has to be put on the table. Above all, Uncle Sam always gets more than his fair share via the taxes. In those tough times the family scraped to make the payments on the farm. When Mr. Banker stopped in the summer of the drought everyone knew there was a problem. Mary guessed Dad cut a deal and managed to keep the farm.

September was a busy month for celebrations, for the entire family had birthdays. September was also harvesting time for canning fruits and vegetables. In the fall the community held a harvest contest. All the farm ladies canned vegetables for the contest. Not to brag much, but Mom canned the best tomatoes and sweet cucumber pickles. She won first prize and was the envy of the ladies. She was a great cook all the way around.

In fact, she cooked in large quantities daily for a threshing crew during harvest time. The smells of breakfast were divine. Bacon was sizzling, along with sausages, potatoes, fried eggs, and pancakes. In addition, hot homemade biscuits were served with churned butter and honey.

Most Sundays Mom made our favorite meal, consisting of chicken and dumplings, garden salad with spicy dressing and hot bread. Grandma usually killed the old red rooster because Mom did not have the heart or the stomach to carry out this particular chore. Some Sundays company came to visit the family and shared the meal. Dad informed all of the kids ahead of time to mind their manners when company arrived. They knew they had to follow Dad's instructions. One time when company arrived the dog ran out and greeted them. Spot jumped on the guest's knees. Dad scolded Spot and told him to get down. Spot then laid down.

During the hot summer days Mom ran a fan when we finally got electricity. It felt so good to have the breeze blow across Mary's sweaty brow on hot sunny days. Gramps called these days dog days. They came once a year in July and August. During this hot spell sometimes the family gathered around and made ice cream. The ice bucket cooled their hands.

Grandma and her friends from church helped out by darning socks and mending clothes when Mom got very ill for a spell. Thank God for Grandmas and good friends. Mom always said she was so lucky to have a kind family.

We lived a mile-and-a-half away from a trout farm. Trout ran from late May through August. Dan and Don loved to fish and sometimes we pan-fried their fresh-caught trout with Mom's special breading. Dad didn't like the trout because he hated to pick out the bones; he also did not like the smell of fish frying because the odor stayed in the house for a long time.

At the end of summer the children returned to the little one-room schoolhouse. Bobbie Joe liked to dunk Mary's pigtails into the inkwell. That was not a fun prank for Mary. One day the teacher caught Bobbie and that was the end of his pranks. He had to write 1,000 times, "I must not dunk Mary's pigtails in the inkwell ever again." Bobbie had writing cramps. Served him right too!

At the beginning of the school year there was a picnic gathering where every family brought their best dish to pass and the recipe. The picnic table looked so festive. Everyone had a great time.

When the children were in school, Dad hired extra help. Sometimes he would run to the hardware store and pick up nails. Mary and her brothers usually walked two miles to school each day. But when Dad ran the errand and timed it right he gave the kids a ride home.

Most of the time Dad was pretty calm. Every once in a while Dad would lose his temper and get angry, especially when the farm equipment broke down.

Dad also got upset if Mable dropped by looking for Mom. She came over from the near-by farm, and she liked to gossip. Dad sure did not like that too much. Mable did all the talking. Dad could never figure out how Mable knew so much, especially since Mable talked incessantly. Dad just nodded his head as Mable talked and said, "Uh huh." After a few moments of conversation Dad would excuse himself and continue with his chores. He always said he had no patience for people who wasted time gossiping, or loafing for that matter.

October was Mom's favorite month of the year. Indian summer was all too short. Pretty colors appeared with the change of the leaves. They watched the full moon and the morning sunrise. The air was fresh and clear at the farm. The family lived in a big old farmhouse set far back off the road. The house had one big window across part of the front of the house. Dad made a nice root cellar for storage of the food. In back of the house was a small play area for the family even though the kids didn't have much time for playing.

Gramps sometime gave Dad a helping hand when he did not have enough workers. However, Gramps was only too glad to retire from the farm for he felt he was getting too old to do all that hard work. Gramps was special. He was quite a storyteller, and he always liked to tease the grandchildren. He made their lives very interesting as he told tall tales. He did a lot of laughing. He believed that laughter was music to the soul.

In the barn was a picture of Gramps with a big grin holding the ram's horns. He used to boast how he would chase and catch this animal while tickling the ram under the chin. Gramps just had a way of making other people laugh and have fun.

The farm was home to many animals, including dogs and cats. The cats kept the mice down some. Dad had a favorite dog named Cal. Dad's dog chased after the sheep until all the sheep were behind the split rail fence. No one ever had time to paint the fence. As a result the fence was left in its natural state.

In the winter Mom and Grandma made sure all of the kids had plenty of woolen hats, gloves, scarves, and socks to keep them toasty warm. On bitter cold days Mary wore long underwear that often was very scratchy.

Holidays were also special. Christmas was a favorite time for the family. The fragrant smells of cakes, cookies, pies, yams, ham, and chestnuts roasting on the fire made everyone inspect the kitchen to see what was cooking. Besides all the preparations the children knew that the birth of the Christ child was the real meaning of Christmas. The best part of Christmas was the anticipation and excitement of that winter holiday.

Every year the family cut down a fresh, tall, stately Christmas tree that was placed in the parlor room. However one particular year the tree was very crooked and stood rather funny. After completing the decorations, the family left the room to eat supper, and there was a loud crash. The tree had toppled over. Mary and her family managed to put the tree back up once again. Dad tied a thin rope around the middle of the trunk of the tree to secure it into place. The tree held through the season.

Uncle Donald usually paid his respects during the holidays. He was a traveling salesman for stoves. He always tried to talk the folks into purchasing one of those newfangled appliances. Every once in a while Mom would burn a pan of biscuits on the open wood fire. He told her it would be cleaner and safer with one of his stoves.

Winter seemed to be the longest season of the year. Sometimes the snow was far too deep to walk through. It helped to know that spring would arrive once again. Spring was in the air as the daffodils poked their green stems and leaves through the black earth and the first robin appeared in this fresh season. Dan, Don, and Mary couldn't wait for spring. The cows and horses had new young'uns. The horse gave birth to a new foal and a cow to a calf. Mary and the twins named all of the animals.

Those days were wonderful days as everyone enjoyed the cycle of the four seasons. Where has the time gone? It seems like only yesterday. Everything seems so vivid in Mary's mind.

Now the farm is gone—it's only a memory.

Mary retired at West Manor Assisted Living about a year ago. Her whole family came today to celebrate her 90th birthday, including her great-grandchildren. This day filled Mary with invisible baskets of flowers and happiness. Mary silently gave thanks to God for her good life and wonderful family and friends. As she posed for photos with smiles she praised the Lord. What could be better than fond memories?

Chicken and Dumplings

To get the wonderful smells of the Sunday dinner on the farm, make up a batch of chicken and dumplings.

Yield: 12 tasting servings

1	fryer chicken, 3 pounds
2	quarts water
1	cup fresh celery leaves
1	onion, sliced in rings
2	cups self-rising flour
$1/2$	teaspoon salt
$1/4$	cup shortening
$1/4$	cup water
$1/2$	cup butter
1	teaspoon black pepper

In large crockpot, cover chicken with 2 quarts water. Add celery leaves and onion. Cook the chicken and vegetables on high heat until done (4 to 6 hours). Remove chicken and vegetables from pot, reserving chicken broth. Cool chicken. Remove bones, skin, and fat. Cut meat into bite-size pieces. Strain out the onion and celery leaves and discard, reserving the broth.

In medium bowl, combine flour and salt. Cut in shortening until coarse crumbs form. Add $1/4$ cup water and mix well with hands. Bring reserved chicken broth to a slow boil. (Do not boil rapidly.) With floured hands, pinch quarter-size pieces of dough and drop into chicken broth. Gently stir after adding several pinches. Repeat until all dumpling mixture is used. Stir gently. Add butter and pepper. Stir gently again. Allow to simmer 8 to 10 minutes. Slowly stir in reserved chicken pieces. Serve in soup bowls.

I cooked the chicken one day in advance. On the day of the farm story I heated up the broth in a pot on the stove. I demonstrated how to make dumplings, then the residents helped mix them. Some floured their hands and pinched off the dough. The smell and touch of the flour and dough is a great sensory tool. Those on unrestricted diets took a few bites of the chicken and dumplings. The smell of the dumplings cooking brightened many faces in the group.

Sing the song "She'll Be Coming 'Round the Mountain When She Comes" and be sure to include the verses:

"Oh we'll kill the old red rooster when she comes"
"Oh we'll all have chicken and dumplings when she comes"
"She'll be wearing red flannel pajamas when she stays (scratch! scratch!)"

(Yell out "scratch, scratch" as you scratch your arms or legs. Try to get the residents to participate in the song.)

In keeping with the theme of an old-fashioned Sunday dinner, conclude the activity with a prayer of thanks and "Amazing Grace."

Prayer of Thanks

We thank Thee O' Lord
For this bright shiny day
Bless this food and fellowship
Thank you for song
To fill our hearts with joy
For the hour
We praise you
In the name of Jesus.
Amen

Farm Theme Picnic at School

I had a gentleman from my parish make up a barn out of wood that was 27-inches high and 27-inches across. He painted it and labeled it "fun farm." There are 15 doors, each of which is 6-inches deep, 6-inches high and 6-inches wide. There are 5 stalls across and 3 down. I lined each stall with straw. This barn was designed for beanbag-style stuffed animals. I decorated it with animals, brown eggs, and apples with leaves. One item was placed into each barn door area to show off to the residents. I did not fasten the items to each area on purpose so that I could change the scenes. In addition I took the animals out so the people could hold them and feel their texture. The residents could touch the straw.

I purchased fabric depicting farm life with apple and other fruit trees and made it into a tablecloth. The tablecloth also has pictures of tractors, farm equipment, animals, grass, and a pond. I held up the fabric and had the residents pick out various objects by asking them one question at a time: Where is the apple tree? the tractor? farmhouse? This tablecloth is very bright in color. The reaction of the residents was very positive. They enjoyed this exercise.

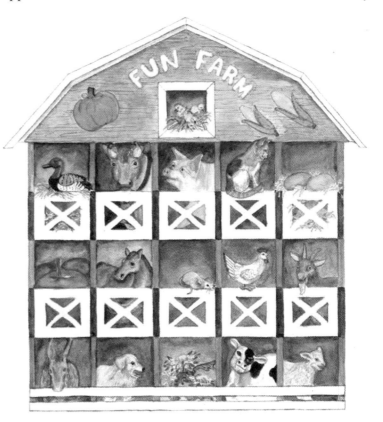

I also passed around a large stuffed animal, a pig. Some of residents enjoyed just holding the pig on their lap. The residents were most impressed with the pig and garden canned goods that I'd also brought. I also displayed a big container of sunflowers. The residents touched the smooth container and the silk flowers that looked so real.

I placed the tablecloth on the table with the farm barn and flowers for display. I passed a picture of a fancy picnic around. The colors of this picture also caught their eye. We discussed what types of foods could be served at a picnic. I asked how many ever attended a picnic. Some could remember and also tell the fun they had with their family. The group sang or hummed with the following songs representing summer and fall. We made ice cream with the residents with the assistance of the staff.

Old-Fashioned Vanilla Ice Cream

Yield: 2 quarts

      2   quarts cream
1 $^1/_2$ cups sugar
      2   teaspoons vanilla
       Rock salt and ice

Set up the ice cream maker according to manufacturer's directions. Pour the cream, sugar, and vanilla into the container, and place the container into the ice cream bucket. Fill the outside bucket with ice and rock salt. Alternate the ice and rock salt to cover the outside of the inside container holding the cream, sugar, and vanilla. Allow to stand for 3-5 minutes before turning slowly. Give the residents a chance to turn the handle. The staff may have to finish turning the handle. Some facilities have electric ice cream makers. The hand-turned ice cream maker becomes quite a conversation piece.

After the ice cream gets started play music and sing while people help make ice cream. I played songs with references to farm animals, frogs, and worms. Serve ice cream with coffee at the end of the program.

"In My Merry Oldsmobile"

"In the Shade of the Old Apple Tree"

"I Scream You Scream"

"Summertime"

"In the Good Old Summertime"

"I Love Paris"

"Ida"

"School Days"

"Rosie O'Grady"

"My Wild Irish Rose"

"When You Wore a Tulip"

"Lavender's Blue"

"Roses Are Red, Violets Are Blue"

"Tie a Yellow Ribbon Around the Old Oak Tree"

"The Chicken Dance"

"Turkey in the Straw"

"Get Along Little Dogies"

"Frog Went A'Courting"

"Glow Worm"

"Mule Skinner Blues"

"Rawhide"

Chapter 17:

SEPTEMBER

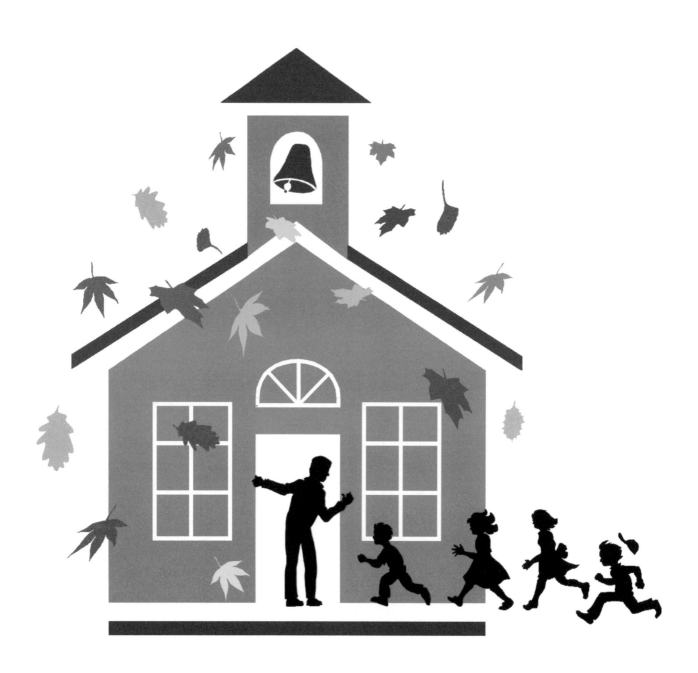

Reminiscing: School Days

Supplies needed:

> School bell.
> Picture of an old schoolhouse.

Ask these questions: Where did you attend grade school? Was it at a one-room school? What did you like about a one-room school? What subject did you like the most? What did you do at recess? Do you remember your teacher's name? What were your fondest memories? Did anyone ever dunk a classmate's pigtails in the inkwell?

Fall Garden Project

A resident's son donated a box of assorted tulip bulbs to the facility. In early September before it got too chilly we brought the residents outside to plant tulips. We showed them the colors on the box of bulbs and talked about how to plant a tulip. We showed the residents the bulb and pointed out the difference between the top and the bottom. We cut apart one of the bulbs for the residents to feel and see the inside.

I told the residents that when I was a little girl I had planted tulips; unfortunately, I planted them bottom side up. In the spring the tulips never came up. I told them we needed to put the bottom side of the tulip toward the ground. We dug holes, reading aloud the package directions, step by step. We placed one bulb per hole. The residents took turns putting water in each hole. We then covered the tulip bulbs with dirt.

In the spring the tulips bloomed. We wheeled the residents back out to the courtyard and played a game. We took them around the courtyard to count the tulips. Next we counted the number of red, yellow, pink, and white tulips.

We served coffee and juice and snacks. The residents had fun and enjoyed seeing, smelling, and touching the tulips; plus they had the extra bonus of the fresh air. This simple activity brought such joy for the moment to each participating resident.

Note: *We monitored one Alzheimer's patient who put everything in her mouth. That is one of the reasons it is so important to know the habits and actions of each resident participating in a group activity.*

Fall Project: A Walk Through Nature

Supplies needed: A selection of tree and shrub branches. I brought:

1 branch of catalpa leaves.
1 branch with apples and leaves.
1 branch of raspberry canes and leaves.
1 branch of crab apple leaves.
1 branch of river birch leaves.
A piece of the birch bark.
1 branch of sumac leaves.
1 branch of silver maple leaves.
1 branch of crimson maple leaves.
1 branch of pin oak leaves.
1 branch of cherry leaves.
1 branch of dogwood leaves.
1 branch of locust leaves.
1 branch of burning bush.
1 branch of green ash.
1 branch of mountain ash.
1 branch of weeping willow leaves.
1 branch of ginkgo leaves.
1 branch of grape leaves.
1 picture of fall leaves to show the color changes.

Present these branches and leaves to the group one at a time. Let each resident touch them and smell the fruit and leaves and the bark of each branch. Point out the shapes of the leaves and fruit. Some can identify the name of the fruit and leaves on the branch. The maple leaf is the one leaf most residents can identify.

For six straight months I went to the same facility, doing sensory and music therapy. One gentleman was always placed around the round table as part of a small group. He watched and listened to the program but never verbally responded. But the day we did this activity was very different. As I talked about the leaves and fruits he suddenly yelled out, "Persimmons! Persimmons! Persimmons! My mother told me never to eat persimmons. There is a male and a female. You just don't know what is good or bad. Some persimmons are poisonous! It is better not to eat any to be safe!"

I stopped what I was doing and bent down by this resident and said, "So you know all about persimmons." He replied, "Yes," I thanked him for that wonderful information.

The activity assistant was pouring juice at this time. She set her container down and broke into a smile. She said, "Did you hear what he said?" It was a moment of joy. You just don't know what will trigger a memory. It was a big bonus for all of us involved in this program. It made my day for this was a major breakthrough.

Show pictures of the various leaves showing the change of colors as you sing songs pertaining to fall:

"I Love Paris"

"Autumn Leaves"

"Kumbaya"
(Fall is here my Lord, Kumbaya, summer is gone my Lord, Kumbaya)

"She'll Be Comin 'Round the Mountain"
(She'll be coming round the mountain in the fall, She'll be carrying pretty leaves when she comes)

"Michael Row the Boat Ashore"
(Michael row the boat ashore in the fall)

"He's Got the Whole World In His Hands"
(He's got the whole fall in His hands)

Note: *The songs that have notes or words repeated is good for jogging an Alzheimer's patient's memory.*

Leaf Art Project

Supplies needed:

> $8^{1}/_{2}$ x 11-inch paper.
> Maple leaves (1 for each person in the group).
> Paint in fall colors.
> Small paint rollers (1 for each color paint).
> Plastic or styrofoam plates.

Press each leaf flat. Lay the leaf on the copy paper. Pour a small amount of paint onto a plate. (Let the resident pick out the color of paint he/she wishes to use.) Load the roller with paint and paint over the leaf on the paper. The background will be filled in and the leaf will be white to show the shape.

Another option: Take paint in several fall colors and splatter on one half of the $8^{1}/_{2}$ x 11-inch paper. Fold the paper in half and blot the paint on the other half. Open the sheet and there will be colors of fall.

I did the branch and singing project in one hour. The art project should be at a separate time or day, repeating the songs if you wish.

Country Fall Harvest Day

Supplies needed:

> Red tomatoes.
> Green tomatoes.
> Onion.
> Fresh chives.
> Zucchini.
> Yellow squash.

Pass the vegetables around to the group and talk about a vegetable garden. Since I grew all of the above vegetables I also brought in the actual plant and leaves that are associated with each vegetable. The residents enjoyed seeing the vegetable attached to the vine. I also left some dirt on the vegetables. It gave them a feeling of being out in their gardens. One group member said that his mother always had a big garden. He could remember her canning lots of tomatoes.

Harvest Vegetable Blend

Yield: 12 servings for tasting

$1/4$	cup margarine
2	red tomatoes, cut into wedges
2	green tomatoes, cut into wedges
1	large green pepper, cut into strips
1	onion sliced into rings
$1/2$	cup chopped fresh chives
1	small zucchini, sliced
1	yellow squash, quartered
	Black pepper
$1/2$	teaspoon garlic seasoning
$1/4$	teaspoon premium blend table spice
1	teaspoon pasta sprinkle

Melt margarine in a large skillet over medium heat. Add red and green tomatoes, green pepper, onion, chives, zucchini, and squash to the skillet. Add pepper, garlic seasoning, premium blend table spice and pasta sprinkle. Saute vegetables 8-10 minutes or until cooked through and tender. Do not overcook.

Note: *If you do not want to take the time to cook all of these vegetables just make fried green tomatoes. However, the residents will enjoy watching and smelling the variety of vegetables.*

You can substitute 2 tablespoons olive oil and 3 tablespoons water for the margarine.

Fried Green Tomatoes, Version I

2   tablespoons margarine

3   green tomatoes, cut into wedges

    garlic seasoning

2   teaspoons pasta sprinkle

Melt margarine in a medium skillet over medium heat. Add tomatoes, garlic seasoning, and pasta sprinkle. Fry tomatoes for 4-5 minutes or until tender, turning occasionally.

Fried Green Tomatoes, Version II

Yield: 15-18 slices

2 cups vegetable oil

3 green tomatoes

1 1/2 cups buttermilk

2 eggs

1 teaspoon salt, divided

1 teaspoon black pepper, divided

1/2 cup self-rising flour, divided

1/2 teaspoon garlic seasoning (optional)

Heat oil to 350 degrees in a large heavy skillet or electric frying pan. Slice tomatoes 1/4 inch thick. Mix buttermilk and eggs in a bowl. Add 1/2 teaspoon each of the salt and pepper and 1 tablespoon of the flour. Mix well. Place tomato slices in the buttermilk mixture. Mix remaining flour, salt and pepper in a separate bowl. Toss the tomato slices in flour mixture. Place in the hot oil, in batches to avoid overcrowding, and fry until golden brown and crisp, turning 2 to 3 times while frying. Drain on paper towels. Serve immediately, sprinkled with garlic seasoning if desired.

Make sure that every group participant can smell the food. Also let them smell the spices used for cooking the vegetables. Many of the residents talked about making fried green tomatoes when they were at home, especially those who lived in the South.

Musical Accompaniment

Play country western songs on tape or with a guitar, piano, or accordion. Have residents sing along.

"Hey Good Lookin'"
What ya got cookin'?
How's about cookin' somethin' up with me?
Hey sweet baby, don't you think maybe
We could find us a brand new recipe.
I got a hot rod Ford and a two dollar bill and I know a spot right over the hill.
There's soda pop and the dancing's free,
So if you wanna have fun come along with me!

Conclude the program with other country western songs:

"Green Green Grass of Home"
"For the Good Times"
"Jambalaya"
"True Grit"
"King of the Road"
"Crazy"

Fall Is In The Air

Supplies needed: A variety of harvest items. I brought:
Scarecrow.
Soybean plant.
Sorghum plant.
1 apple tree branch.
1 grapevine with grapes.
2 sunflowers with seeds.
1 raspberry cane.
1 asparagus fern.
1 bunch of cornstalks with dried corn and Indian corn.
Chrysanthemums.
Assortment of gourds.
1 small white pumpkin and 1 orange pumpkin.

Scarecrow: Hold up the scarecrow and ask if anyone knows what it is. One woman knew immediately that it was a scarecrow. "I grew up on the farm," she said. "My dad had scarecrows in his fields." Pass the scarecrow around and let residents feel the roughness of the burlap garb. Talk about how the scarecrow looks and his style of hat. Show off his face and smile and eyes.

Soybean plant: Pull off a couple of soybeans. Let the residents feel the furriness of the outside of a soybean. Let them see the whole plant and touch the texture of the leaves and stem. Break open the pod and let the residents inspect the bean.

Sorghum plant: Sorghum syrup is made from the stems of the plant. Pass around the plant. Tell them that sorghum stems are cooked up and made into syrup for pancakes. In the north most people will have to buy sorghum at a specialty food store.

Apple tree branch: Inspect the shape of the leaves. Cut open the apple and show the seeds. They can smell the apple.

Grapevine with leaves: Cut open the grapes and let the residents smell them. Talk about the shape and texture of the leaf.

Sunflowers: Take some seeds out of the sunflower and hold the seeds in your hand for the residents. Let them touch and smell the flower.

Raspberry cane: Let the residents feel the rougher texture of these leaves.

Asparagus fern: With the residents' permission, use the fern to stroke the residents lightly on their arms to feel the feather-soft texture.

Dried corn: Let them feel the softness of the cornsilk and also the hardness of the fall corn. Let them feel the corn husks. Show the colors of the Indian corn. One of the residents saw the vibrant colors of the Indian corn and yelled, "It is just beautiful."

Chrysanthemums: The mums in bright colors get the resident's attention. They like to smell the freshly cut flowers and see the vivid colors.

Gourds: Pass the gourds around and let the residents feel the nubby texture of the gourds. Also show the colors of yellow, orange, and deep green.

The sight and smell of these items elicited fond memories. When I passed the grapevine and grapes, a resident said, "I used to have those in my backyard. I made grape jelly and juice." Another resident remembered making applesauce with the apples from her backyard. Someone else said, "Our family planted sunflowers special for the birds. That way they could have the seeds for food."

Grape Juice

        6   cups water
        3   pounds Concord grapes
    1$^1/_2$ cups sugar

Take the grapes off the vine and wash. Place drained grapes into the crockpot with water. Add the sugar and stir. Cook on high heat for about two hours. Mash grapes with a potato masher during cooking. Stir every half hour. Pour mixture into a sieve, pressing the pulp to extract all the liquid. Cool the juice.

The smell of the juice cooking really alerts the resident's senses.

Reminiscing: Apples

Supplies needed:

    A variety of apples.
    Apple peeler.
    Apple slicer.
    Apple corer.
    Pie pan.

Discussion questions: Can you identify the different kinds of apples? Which one is the juiciest? Which is sweet? Which is sour? Which is best for baking? Which apple do you like the best? What utensils did you use to prepare apples? What are some of the apple dishes you've made? (Pie, kuchen, applesauce, apple crisp, apple dumplings, apple cake, apple brown betty, apple cobbler, caramel apples, candy apples, juice, cider.) Why will an apple a day keep the doctor away? (Contains high fiber, reduces serum cholesterol levels, decreases cancer risk.) Apples are naturally sweet and fun to eat! Apples can be crunchy, juicy, sweet, or tart.

Reminiscing: Canning

Supplies needed:

      Hot water bath canner.

      Food mill.

      Lids and rings.

      Jars.

      Jar lifter.

      Measuring spoons and cups.

      Timer.

      Long-handled wooden spoons.

      Jar funnel.

      Hot pads.

      Warm applesauce for tasting.

Pass around and display these items as you reminisce about canning. Questions for discussion:

Have you ever canned? Who helped you can? What did you like best about canning? What is your favorite thing to can? How many pounds of apples are needed to fill a one-quart jar? ($2^1/_2$-3 pounds.) About how much does a bushel of apples weigh? (48 pounds.) How do you know if a jar is sealed? (Most jars will seal with a "pop" noise) How long does it take to seal and cool a sealed jar? (12 to 24 hours.) What did you can? (Juices, jams, jellies, preserves, marmalades, butters, conserves, fruits, sauces, chutneys, tomatoes, pickles, relishes, soups, meats, poultry, and seafood.) What kind of problems did you have when you canned? (Fruit floating in jars, browning of fruit, air bubbles.) Did you leave the peeling on or off when you made applesauce? What time of year did you can? What did it smell like? Did you have a summer kitchen?

Apple Fest

I purchased a book called *Apples* by Roger Yepsen. This book has a great deal of information about apples. It has many pictures of apples and information on the varieties to add interest to the program. It is an excellent book for not only group activity but one-on-one. I read the book and used some of the facts to create a story describing apples. I purchased apples from an apple orchard and showed the residents some of the varieties of apples in the discussion. I cut the apples for tasting and we made an apple recipe of their choice. In addition, we played songs about apples and remembered apple sayings.

Songs:
"Cherry Pink and Apple Blossom White"
"Don't Sit Under the Apple Tree"
"Apples and Bananas"
"Apple Blossom Wedding"
"Apple Jump"
"Apple Sass Rag"
"Apple Strudel"
"Ida"
"Cindy"
"In the Shade of the Old Apple Tree"

Sayings:

Let the residents complete the saying with "apple."

1. She is the _____ of my eye.

2. An _____ a day will keep the doctor away.

3. _____s are sweet and tart and everything nice.

4. _____s grow on trees.

5. Ida was sweeter than _____ cider.

Applesauce

Yield: 1 pound applesauce (6 servings)

6	medium cooking apples
4	cups water
$1/3$	cup sugar
$1/2$	teaspoon apple pie spice

Cut apples into quarters. Leave on peels. Core apples. Place into a medium saucepan; add water. Cover pan with a lid and bring to a boil. Cook until apples are tender, 6-8 minutes. Drain off excess water. Place apples into a sieve and strain the applesauce. Discard the peels. Add sugar and apple pie spice to the applesauce. Stir until well blended. Place into a bowl, cover and refrigerate.

Sweet and Sour Red Cabbage

Yield: 4 servings

$1/2$	pound red cabbage
$1/4$	cup margarine
2	cooking apples, peeled, cored, and sliced
2	cups water
$1/4$	cup vinegar
$1/2$	cup sugar
$1/2$	teaspoon salt
$1/4$	teaspoon pepper

Cut cabbage into bite-size pieces. Melt margarine in large skillet. Add cabbage, apples, water, vinegar, sugar, salt, and pepper. Stir together. Simmer until cabbage is tender.

While the red cabbage was cooking, the smell raised eyebrows and sparked conversation in the room. Once the cabbage and apple dish was cooked I passed it around for the group to smell. One participant spontaneously put her hand into the bowl and picked out an apple slice. She devoured the apple with a gleeful smile, savoring every bite. It was a joy to watch her.

Haddie's Apple Story

Grandma was very particular about having just the right apple for her favorite apple dishes. She explained that there are hundreds of apple varieties. There just ain't nothin' like a good old-fashioned cookin' apple like the McIntosh for making a delicious pie. She did admit that lard in the pie crust also helped complete the great taste. Grandma rendered the lard but Haddie could not remember how Grandma tackled the process. Haddie just knew Grandma's method for baking a pie resulted in some good eating. Grandma was of a staunch Dutch background. She swore that an apple a day would keep the doctor away. But she also added that an onion a day would keep everyone away. Haddie said that is probably why she never took to eating many onions in her life.

Haddie was the apple of her dad's eye. She could do no wrong in his estimation. She was the girl that represented sugar and spice and everything nice. Dad also said that Haddie had the most knowledge of apples. She knew her apples, all right. "A red Delicious is so beautiful and great for eating," Haddie exclaimed. She decided that the group of farm visitors should just cut one open and taste it to be sure. The group enjoyed the tiny bites of this juicy apple. Smiling faces showed a round of approval as they taste-tested this red beauty.

A huge pot sat on the wood fire filled with cooking apples with a scent of cinnamon. Grandma strained off the juice and turned this delightful dish into applesauce. She knew how to sweeten and add just the right spice to please our taste buds. Gramps liked to just pick and shine an apple on his bright, red-plaid flannel shirt. He enjoyed a fresh apple while doing a few of his chores on the farm. He never passed up Grandma's applesauce or pie. Gramps also enjoyed a little cider moonshine. He said it kept him healthy. Grandma begged to differ. "Oh well," said Haddie.

At any rate, cider was a very popular beverage back in those good old days. Apples were fermented easily. Uncle Herman got right down to business and wasted no time as he made his favorite apple brandy. He didn't share his concoction either. Uncle Herman had to curtail his applejack making when the Temperance Act went through the country. Folks say in one county alone, there was distilled about 310 gallons of apple brandy. Apple cider was introduced to America by the English. Cider was a healthy beverage served at mealtime. Uncle Herman said that it started way back in Pennsylvania in the 1700s. The farm families would put up 15 to 40 barrels of cider every fall. The horse was the power for the fruit grinder.

Then there was cider soup that was thickened with flour and sweet cream, and served with croutons. Auntie Mamime insisted you must know your apples to make good apple cider. There are two kinds of cider apples: sweet and tart. She listed her favorite varieties: "Red Delicious, Golden Delicious, Cortland, Rome Beauty, Empire, Winesap, Jonathan, Wealthy, and McIntosh."

Haddie said that as she grew up and raised her family she could go to the supermarket and buy apples. However, they just were not as good as getting them from the farm or going to an apple orchard. Haddie liked the Spartan because she remembered this apple to be firm and crisp. "Just smell the aroma and see the snow-white flesh!" she exclaimed. "It reminds me of the McIntosh that Grandma swore by."

"Oh my!" Haddie said, "Just look at that big Wolverine apple."

"It is huge," I said. "How do you know that apple?"

Haddie said, "I know my apples. My dad taught me the facts. Besides, it is my favorite fruit."

One of the apples I learned about that grows in Wisconsin is the Wolverine which grows from seed. It was noted way back in 1875 along the banks of the Wolf River. My brother and I canoed on the Wolf River and tasted a few.

The Rome Beauty was known before the Civil War. This apple has a long shelf life and is a beautiful red color with a nice shape. It is crisp, firm, and mildly tart. Harvest usually happens from late September into November.

The Winesap has real character. It is firm and very juicy with a sweet-sour contrast. It is a great apple for making cider, applesauce, and pie. It was an important cider apple starting back in 1817. Cider vinegar was another product extracted from this apple.

After we talked about all of these apples, I prepared some apple dishes.

Apple Cake

Yield: one 9x13-inch cake

Brown sugar topping:

$1/2$ cup butter, softened
$1/2$ cup packed brown sugar
$1/2$ cup oatmeal
$1/2$ cup flour

Cake:

1   white cake mix (follow the directions on the box for amounts of water, oil and eggs)
1   teaspoon ground cloves
1   teaspoon apple pie spice
3   medium cooking apples, peeled, cored and diced

For topping, in a small bowl beat butter. Add brown sugar, oatmeal and flour. Beat until creamy. Set aside.

Preheat oven to 350 degrees. Prepare the cake mix according to directions on the box and add cloves, apple pie spice, and apples to the batter. Beat until smooth. Place cake batter into a 9x13-inch cake pan.

Drop topping on top of the cake batter at random until entire cake has drops of topping. This topping is not to be spread over the top nor does it have to cover the entire cake. Bake for 45-50 minutes or until toothpick inserted in center of cake comes out clean. Cool cake. Frost with non-dairy whipped topping. Cut into small squares for tasting.

Apple Strudel

Yield: 9x13-inch strudel

1/2	box (8 ounces) phyllo dough
1/4	cup margarine, melted
1	can (1 pound 14 ounces) apple pie filling

Glaze:

1/2	cup powdered sugar
1/2	teaspoon almond extract
1/2	teaspoon salt
1 1/2	teaspoons water

Thaw phyllo dough; keep covered. Brush margarine over bottom of 9x13-inch pan and line with one layer of phyllo sheets, overlapping if necessary. Brush with melted butter. Add 3 more layers of phyllo sheets, brushing each with more melted butter. Pour apple pie filling over phyllo dough. Cover filling with a layer of phyllo sheets. Brush with melted butter. Repeat as with bottom crust, using remaining phyllo sheets. Brush top sheet with melted butter. Cover well and refrigerate overnight.

Preheat oven to 400 degrees. Bake for 20-25 minutes or until golden brown.

In a small bowl, mix powdered sugar, almond extract, salt, and water to form a glaze. Drizzle over strudel as soon as it comes out of the oven.

Note: *You can substitute cherry pie filling for the apple filling, if desired.*

Tip: *You can purchase phyllo dough at the grocery store in a 1-pound box, containing approximately twenty 14x8-inch sheets. The sheets are paper-thin and fragile; keep unused dough covered with waxed paper and a damp towel over the waxed paper or in a plastic bag while working to keep it from drying out.*

Apple Pie

Fresh apple pie is a favorite pie of most folks. Apple pie was served as far back as 1630 in New England. The folks used up their apples from the orchards. It was a delicious treat enjoyed by all the townspeople. Baseball and apple pie are considered all-American. Well, at least apple pie is unanimously liked. A tart cooking apple is a must for making an apple pie. Cortland, McIntosh, Granny Smith, Wealthy, or Rome Beauty are good pie apples. My favorite are McIntosh and Granny Smith. Granny Smiths are green apples that are very tart. McIntosh apples are red and firm. Avoid using a Delicious apple. It is a good eating apple but doesn't hold up well in pies. For a 9 x 1-inch pie, I use 5 large apples (6 ounces each).

For this activity, you should have a display of the cooking apples. I passed the apple varieties and talked about them. Some of the participants were still able to peel apples. We worked with them to do so. One lady could not peel or core apples any longer but she could cut the apples into quarters and slice the quarters into thin slices. She was very proud that she could participate in the pie-making assembly. It made her feel important and needed.

I have a friend who uses three varieties of apples in her pie, Cortland, Granny Smith, and McIntosh. Her pies are delicious.

Basic Pie Crust

Yield: 1 double crust for 9- or 10-inch pie.

3	cups flour
$3/4$	teaspoon salt
1	teaspoon sugar
$1^1/4$	cups shortening
1	teaspoon vinegar
1	egg, beaten
$1/3$	cup ice cold water

In a large bowl, mix flour, salt, and sugar. Blend shortening into flour mixture until pea-size crumbs form. Add vinegar and egg to water and blend into flour mixture until dough holds together. Divide dough into two balls, one slightly larger than the other. Roll out larger ball between two pieces of waxed paper, or on a floured countertop. Line a pie pan with the dough. Roll out smaller ball for the top of the pie and set aside.

Apple Pie

3/4	cup plus 1 tablespoon sugar, divided
3/4	teaspoon cinnamon
2	tablespoons cornstarch
1	tablespoon lemon juice
4	cups apples, peeled, cored, thinly sliced
2	tablespoons butter or margarine
	Dough for 1 double crust
1	egg
1	tablespoon milk

Preheat oven to 425 degrees for an aluminum pie pan and 400 degrees for a glass pie pan. In a small bowl, mix 3/4 cup of the sugar, cinnamon, and cornstarch together. In a large bowl, pour lemon juice over sliced apples. Toss gently to coat; pat apples dry. Blend cinnamon-sugar mixture into apples. Place apples into unbaked pie crust. Dot with butter. Cover with top piecrust. Seal pie crusts together and cut slits in top to allow steam to escape. Mix together egg and milk; brush over top of crust. Sprinkle remaining 1 tablespoon sugar over center of crust.

Bake pie for 15 minutes. Turn temperature down to 375 degrees for aluminum pie pan or 350 degrees for glass. Bake 35-45 minutes longer or until crust is golden brown and apples are tender.

Pie-making Tips

When I was in school, I learned that I should use two thirds of the dough for the bottom crust and one third for the top. See if the residents can tell the difference in the size of the ball of dough. I also rolled out the dough in between two pieces of waxed paper by dampening the countertop and placing the waxed paper on the damp surface. Place the dough on the waxed paper and place a second sheet of waxed paper over the dough. Roll out the dough to fit the size of the pie pan. Remove the top sheet of waxed paper and place the dough into the pan. Peel off the second sheet of waxed paper. Repeat for the top crust.

Use extra dough to make pie stick treat. Many remembered doing this activity with their own children. It brings back fond memories for the residents.

Pie Stick Treat

Roll out extra dough. Sprinkle cinnamon and sugar over the dough. Cut into strips. Place onto an ungreased cookie sheet. Bake at 375 degrees for 5-8 minutes or until golden brown. For a different shape you can twist the pie sticks or cut out shapes such as hearts from the dough.

Note: You might ask the residents how many of them rolled out their pie dough on a floured board with a floured rolling pin.

Chapter 18:

OCTOBER

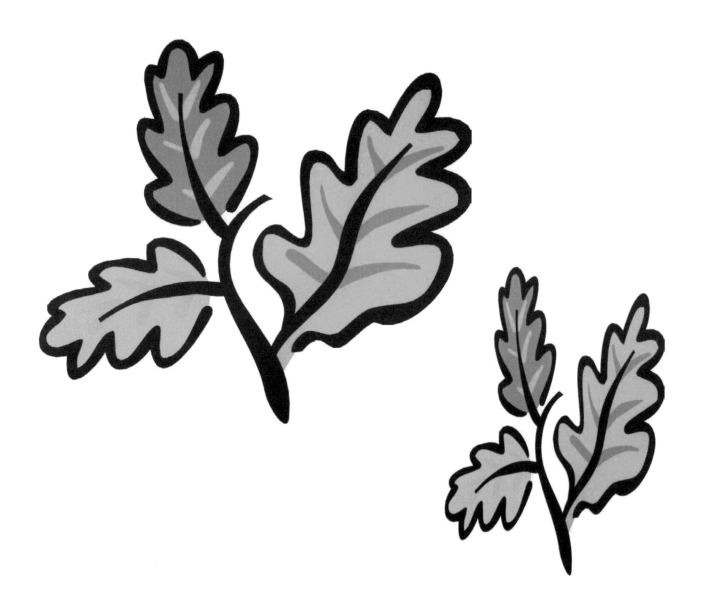

Autumn Harvest Celebration

I started the program by asking, "Who in here likes to eat?" Almost everyone agreed that it was fun to taste various foods. I then led into my story about harvest celebrations.

Parched by dog days and exhausted with working from sunrise to dusk in the heat, early Americans welcomed and applauded the coming of cooler weather with autumn harvest celebrations. Many were relieved to see cooler temperatures in the fall. Autumn is a special season because colors of the trees change. In late fall grass becomes yellow brown and frost covers the ground. Indeed, Jack Frost is showing his cool spirit. However, late autumn days can be very brisk and challenging to stay warm. In the old days during the autumn many people chopped wood, repaired their houses, and stored food for the long hard winter ahead. Wheat stood up in tied bundles in a stately manner in farmers' fields across the nation. It was a wonderful time to celebrate the beauty of the fruitful crops. It was a time to reflect on the success of the farmers.

Amish farmers work long hard hours growing crops without machinery and modern-day farm techniques. Today vegetables can be grown in greenhouses and food is produced year-round. Fall is apple-picking time. Machinery is not used to pick the fruit.

Food festivals were a must to celebrate a great harvest. People feared that if their crops failed they might starve to death. So it was very important to work hard to grow their crops to perfection. The entire family, friends, and neighbors worked together with great pride. That pride is what built this great nation called America.

People, for thousand of years across the globe, have grown crops and have celebrated their success at the time of harvest. Bavarian Oktoberfest in Germany first started in 1723 to celebrate the king's marriage. It is celebrated each year in Germany while people stuff themselves with a variety of sausages, breads, desserts, and beer. In many Asian countries, rice harvest takes place in the autumn. They also pick apples. In that particular climate, harvest begins in the spring and ends in the late fall. The workers celebrate with singing and dancing and having a party with workers and friends.

Britain has several harvest festivals. People parade in suits with multicolored pearl buttons on their garments. These people are called the pearly king and queen as they wear the traditional costume covered with pearls. This tradition started in the nineteenth century in London. Fishermen also enjoy participating in harvest festivals. Many Christians attending special services brought their harvest to the event.

In Africa, people celebrate harvest festivals by wearing masks to tell stories of the spirits that control the harvest of their crops. They dance to African music and feast on their crops.

Thanksgiving is a traditional family day celebrated in America, on the fourth Thursday in November, with a menu including turkey, yams, potatoes, cranberries, and pumpkin pie. Canada celebrates Thanksgiving in October.

The Japanese celebrate the autumn crop of rice. They will not eat the rice until they have held a celebration in honor of the spirits for protecting the crop during the growing season. At the celebration, part of the harvest would be delivered to the sacred altar to give thanks for the success of the harvest.

There are also tropical harvest festivals in Southeast Asia. This region has three seasons—dry, rainy, and cold. The rainy season begins in July and ends at the end of October. The people then celebrate Onam to rejoice for the end of the rainy season. The children gather a variety of flowers to be woven into colorful mats. They are rewarded with new clothes. The people clean their homes and decorate the floors. Once the preparation is completed they go to the temple to give thanks for a prosperous harvest. They then have a big feast with rice, vegetables, spiced curry, and sweet puddings. Boat races along the lagoon become part of the activity for the day. These long boats have carvings of birds' tails and snakes' heads. Think of how wonderful it is to celebrate in thanksgiving for the harvest of good food in the world.

Serve non-alcoholic beer and sodas with pretzels.

Play a variety of polkas in honor of German Oktoberfest and end the program with the song "When Autumn Leaves Start to Fall."

Wheelchair Dancing

I danced with the residents in their wheelchairs. I have a CD with a variety of polkas. Their three favorite polkas are "The Beer Barrel Polka," "In Heaven There Is No Beer," and "Just Because." I also played the "Tick Tock" and "Rain Rain" polkas. They enjoyed watching me do the bellow shakes on the accordion while playing the "Tick Tock" polka.

Bones

Show a picture of a skeleton that you've cut in half horizontally. Lay each piece on the table before the group and get each person to match the two pieces. In my experience, some residents were able to match top to bottom. We helped the residents tape the two pieces together. I made sure each resident in the group had their own picture of a skeleton.

Get the residents to fill in the appropriate body part in the following sentences.

If you don't use your head you will use your _____. (feet)

Milk keeps your _____ healthy. (bones or teeth)

To dance you need to move your _____ and _____ (feet and hips). Plus hold _____ (hands) and then dance _____ to _____. (cheek to cheek)

A tendon named after an ancient Greek warrior in the Trojan War is _____. (Achilles tendon)

Exercise helps the _____ to keep physically fit. (body)

Exercise For Bones

Exercise each body part as you discuss it.

Head: Tilt head back. Tilt head forward. Tilt head to the right side. Tilt head to the left side. Rotate head gently in a circular motion: chin to chest, then right ear to right shoulder, head back, left ear to left shoulder.

Jawbone: Open mouth wide and close 5 times. Yawn wide.

Collarbone: Take your right hand and touch your collarbone 5 times. Take your left hand

and touch your collarbone 5 times.

Elbow: Bend your right elbow twice. Bend your left elbow twice. Bend both elbows, giving yourself a cross-your-heart squeeze.

Wrists: Shake your wrists and hands. Using a small rubber ball, put ball in one hand and squeeze ball; switch hands.

Hands: Shake hands with the person next to you.

Pelvic bone: Wiggle in your chair.

Foot: Pick up your left foot and set it down. Pick up your right foot and set it down.

Ribs: Touch your ribs.

The purpose of this is to get the residents to become aware of their body parts, to exercise, and follow one-step directions.

Singing:

(To the tune of "Kumbaya")

> Thank you Lord for my bones,
>
> Thank you Lord for my feet, (wiggle toes).
>
> Thank you Lord for my legs, (lift legs).
>
> Thank you Lord for my hands, (wiggle fingers or put hands together in
>
>   a prayerful manner or rub hands together).
>
> Thank you Lord for my head, (tap their head).
>
> Thank you Lord for my hips, (hands on hips).
>
> Thank you Lord for my arms, (rock a baby doll in their arms. It gives
>
>   them a sense of need and happiness).
>
> Thank you Lord for my teeth, (show teeth).
>
> Thank you Lord for my ears, (hands over ears).
>
> Thank you Lord for my lips.

Coffee & Tea & Bones & Me (Missing body parts game)

We played a missing body parts game at coffee hour. Play these songs with the residents and some will be able to name the missing body parts.

"When Irish _____ Are Smiling" (eyes).

"Peg O' My _____" (heart).

"Ma, He's Making _____ at Me" (eyes).

"Baby _____" (face).

"Smoke Gets in Your _____" (eyes).

"Dancing _____ to _____" (cheek to cheek).

"Funny _____" (face).

"Five Foot Two, _____ of Blue" (eyes).

"I've Got You Under My _____" (skin).

"My _____ Belongs to Daddy" (heart).

"Dear _____ and Gentle People" (hearts).

"Put Your _____ Around Me Honey" (arms).

"The Curse of the Aching _____" (heart).

"What Do You Want to Make Those _____ at Me For" (eyes).

"Here in My _____" (arms).

"Clap Your _____" (hands).

"When Your _____ Has Turned to Silver" (hair).

"Time on My _____" (hands).

"Full Moon and Empty _____" (arms).

"The Touch of Your _____" (hands).

"Don't Let the Stars Get in Your _____" (eyes).

"Your Cheatin' _____" (heart).

"My _____ Has a Mind of Its Own" (heart).

"I Dream of Jeannie With the Light Brown _____" (hair).

Card Making

Supplies needed:

Glossy card paper, folded in half to 4^1/$_4$"x 5^1/$_2$".

1 set of paints in fall colors.

1 plastic or styrofoam plate.

1 small paint roller.

1 leaf stamp.

Gold paint.

Cover your table with layers of newspaper or an inexpensive plastic tablecloth to protect it from the paint. Pour small amounts of each color of paint onto the plate. Lay card out flat. Roll the roller over the paint. Roll over card until the glossy side of the card is covered with the fall colors. Let the cards sit until paint is dry.

Dab some gold paint on the leaf stamp. Press down on the painted side of the card to get the gold leaf imprint. The card needs to dry thoroughly for about one hour. Do not stack cards while drying.

Tip: *Sell the cards at an arts and crafts fair to raise extra funds for other activities.*

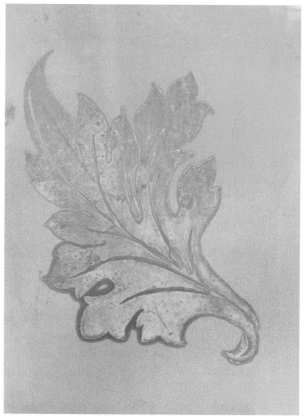

Halloween

Halloween is celebrated on October 31 each year. Halloween is the oldest celebrated holiday. How did Halloween come to be as we know it today?

Many years ago in Europe the Celts worshiped many gods. People thought that witches were real. The Celts thought winter was the season of death. The Celts believed if they dressed up, the spirits would not recognize them and they would not be picked for death. The name Halloween really comes from All Hallows Eve, meaning holy evening (November 1st is All Saints' Day); it was later shortened to Halloween.

Black and orange are the colors commonly associated with Halloween. Black stood for death and night, and orange stood for the harvest and fire to keep the demons away. Witches and brooms, ghosts, black cats, goblins, and bats are all part of Halloween decorations. Witches are seen in pictures with pointed hats, black garb, and flying on a broom. In the past, witches got together in the deep forest at midnight. This gathering was called a sabbat. The most important sabbat was celebrated on Halloween.

There are many stories about witches, especially from Salem, Massachusetts. Witches were persecuted in the late 1600s. Many people believed that witches could turn themselves into cats. They thought black cats had a magical power and even thought cats were spirits.

Carving pumpkins is a Halloween tradition. Families across America carve pumpkins to turn them into jack-o'-lanterns, with a candle placed inside. The Irish immigrants are responsible for bringing their Halloween customs to America and starting the jack-o'-lantern tradition.

The story goes that there was a mean, stingy man named Jack. After he died he was barred from heaven. He then hollowed out a turnip and placed a hot glowing coal inside. He would walk the land at night with his lit turnip. He became known as Jack O'Lantern.

Today people just dress up and go door-to-door and say "trick or treat." It's just a fun night out with friends, family, and neighbors. Many people decorate their front porches and entire homes with Halloween decorations such as scarecrows, skeletons, pumpkins, cornstalks, bales of hay, and fall vegetables. People go on hayrides or to a dance. Some bob for apples. Hot apple cider is a favorite beverage served at Halloween parties.

People enjoy seeing each other in costumes, while others like to hear scary stories, music, and Halloween sound effects to get into the mood of celebrating. Some communities set up a haunted house to raise funds for their favorite charities. In some of the schools, adult day care centers, and nursing homes a prize is given out for the most creative or funniest costume or best decorated window or nurse's station. It all adds up to great fun and conversation to bring joy to all involved in the activity.

One Halloween when I was ten I decided to dress up like a bride. I thought it would be ideal to wear my mother's wedding dress. It would be inexpensive and so exciting to be a bride. I did not ask my mother for permission. I climbed up into the closet and got the dress down. When Mom arrived home from work I was all ready to go trick-or-treating. I asked, "How do you like my costume?" I was much surprised at my mom's reaction. I was instructed, "Take off that dress immediately or else!" I knew she was very upset with me and I immediately took off her wedding dress. I never saw that dress again. I did not go out to trick-or-treat that year. I must admit it was a thrill to try on my mom's dress. I still have a picture of my mom in her beautiful wedding gown. I will always remember that incident and will cherish her picture.

Many residents didn't remember much about getting dressed in costumes and going door-to-door for treats on Halloween, but they enjoy the stories.

One October day I brought my collection of witches to the facility. The residents enjoyed looking at my collection. My favorite witch is almost five feet tall. One of the male residents said, "Boy, is that witch ever ugly!" Another male resident said, "Quiet! That is my girlfriend you're talking about!"

I played Halloween theme music and some polkas on my accordion. I also served cheese and crackers and apple cider.

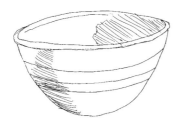 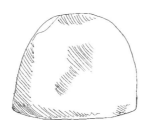 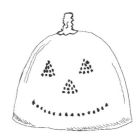

Pumpkin Cake

Preheat oven to 350 degrees. Grease and flour a 2-quart round mixing bowl (this will give the cake its pumpkin shape). Make yellow cake or pumpkin cake batter from a mix, following the directions on the box. Place the cake batter into the bowl. Bake 40-45 minutes or until a toothpick inserted in the center comes out clean. Cool for 5 minutes and invert cake carefully onto a plate.

Frosting:
$1/2$ cup margarine
$1/2$ cup shortening
1 pound powdered sugar
$1/4$-$1/3$ cup water
1 teaspoon almond extract
Few drops each orange and green food coloring
Chocolate chips

Cream margarine and shortening together. Alternately add powdered sugar and $1/4$ - $1/3$ cup water to creamed mixture, ending with powdered sugar. Add almond extract. Beat until smooth and creamy. Reserve $1/2$ cup frosting and color it green. Add orange food coloring to the remainder of the frosting. Frost the cooled pumpkin cake with the orange frosting. Fill a pastry bag with the green frosting, using a very large star tube, and pipe on the stem for the top of the cake. With a toothpick run lines down the side of the cake to make it look like the ridges on a pumpkin. Add a triangle nose, two eyes and a mouth on the pumpkin with the chocolate chips.

The residents can help mix the cake batter and frosting. I demonstrated how to frost and decorate the pumpkin. They enjoyed the activity.

Illustration on How to Make a Halloween Ghost

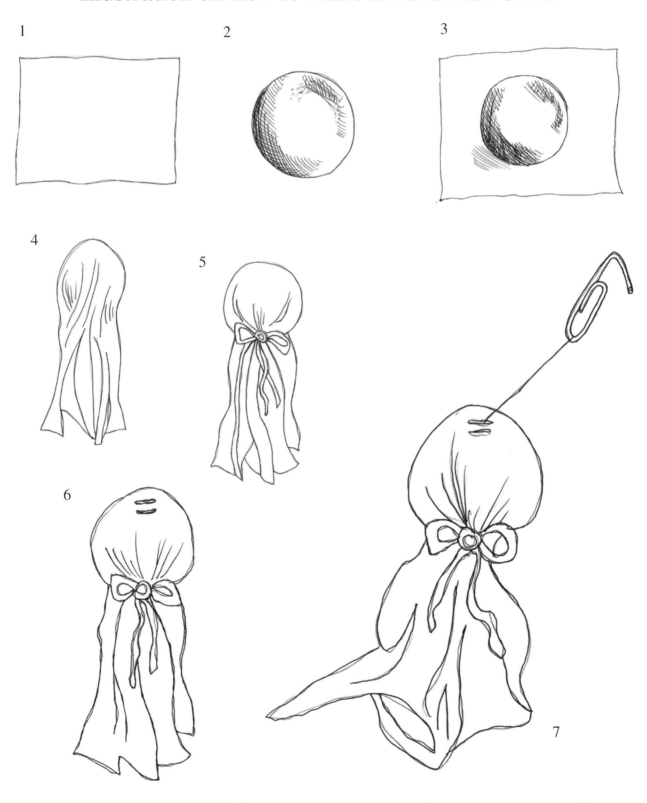

Halloween Ghosts

While making ghosts with the residents in a small group I talked to them about Halloween.

See pictures of each step of this project on opposite page.

Supplies needed for each ghost:

>Cotton or lightweight fabric with Halloween print (Do not use silky material. It will slip and slide. A 30-inch length of material 45-inches wide will make eight 11x15-inch ghosts.)
>1 bag polyester fiberfill.
>1 piece of black or white yarn 36-inches long.
>1 piece of black or white yarn 30-inches long.
>Scotch tape.
>1 paper clip.
>Pinking shears and Scissors.

Cut an 11x15-inch rectangle out of newspaper to make a pattern. Fold fabric in half lengthwise. Lay the newspaper rectangle on the fabric and pin in place. Cut out the rectangle with pinking shears.

Prepare a golf ball-sized ball of polyester fiberfill. Place ball in the center of the material. Fold fabric over the fiberfill to form the ghost's head. Wrap the 36-inch piece of yarn around end of ball to form neck area. Tie yarn once. Wrap yarn around neck three more times and tie again. Tie the remaining yarn into a long bow. Tie a knot in the bow.

Make two $3/8$-inch slits in the middle of the head directly across from each other with a $3/4$-inch space in between the slits. Wrap a $3/4$-inch piece of tape around the end of the 30-inch piece of yarn to form a needle. Pull the yarn through the slit. Get the two ends of the yarn to meet. Tie a knot at the slit. Slide yarn through the paper clip, leaving a few inches of yarn between the paper clip and the ghost's head. Tie a knot to the end of the paper clip and cut off excess yarn. Form a hook at the top of the paper clip. Hang the ghosts from the ceiling, using different lengths of string.

Note: *The activity staff may have to cut out the materials and the yarn pieces. Most of the residents will be able to hold the ball in their hand and work the ball. This is excellent for* *exercise of their fingers. They also enjoy the colors and figures in the material. The residents enjoyed seeing the ghosts hanging up in their lunch area. You can make bigger ghosts, but the size I describe is very easy for the residents to handle.*

Halloween Luncheon

Menu:

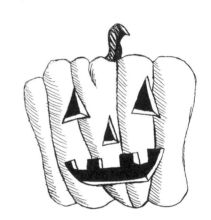

Ginger pumpkin soup
Crab cheese ball and crackers
Cheese and meat tray with condiments
French bread
Breadsticks
Butter
Donuts
Hot apple cider punch
Coffee and milk

Send out invitations one month in advance. Ask for an RSVP. Also put signs around the facility, and publicize the party in the facility's newsletter. The residents helped me chop the vegetables and make the Ginger Pumpkin Soup (see recipe, on opposite page). They also made the crab cheese ball (see recipe, page 248) and arranged crackers in a basket. They mixed the punch ingredients (see recipe, page 248) together and put the holes in the home-made donuts (see recipe, page 248). I fried the donuts away from the residents' reach. They had coffee while they waited for the donuts to cook. They shook the donuts in the bag to coat them with powdered sugar and put them in lined baskets.

Make soup and the cheese ball, set up the cheese and meat tray and carve a pumpkin one day before the party. Set the table with a Halloween tablecloth, napkins, and a centerpiece early in the morning day of the party. Slice French bread and arrange in baskets. Place bread-sticks in baskets. Heat the punch and make the coffee. Arrange the food on the table and serve your guests.

(I would suggest that if young children come to the party, cook hot dogs and serve chips for the kids. Have a few extra just in case the residents would like to have a hot dog.) I found that Saturday is a good day to serve families.

The first- and second-stage Alzheimer's patients really enjoyed this activity. A couple of the third-stage Alzheimer's patients came to the cooking preparation center. They liked watching and smelling the good foods. They enjoyed being in the group. The families are very appreciative and happy to see their loved ones participating in group activities such as cooking.

Ginger Pumpkin Soup

Yield: 12 servings

- $^1/_2$ cup margarine
- $1^1/_4$ cups finely chopped leek
- 1 bunch scallions, finely chopped
- $^1/_3$ cup peeled and finely chopped fresh ginger root
- 1 teaspoon crushed garlic
- 2 cups diced cooked turkey
- 2 cans (16 ounces each) pumpkin
- 1 can (12 ounces) evaporated milk
- 1 cup white wine
- 3 cups chicken broth
- 2 tablespoons brown sugar
- 2 tablespoons freshly squeezed orange juice
- 1 teaspoon white pepper
- 2 teaspoons pasta sprinkle
- Fresh chopped parsley for garnish

On medium heat melt margarine in a skillet. Add leek, scallions, ginger, and garlic. Saute until soft. Add turkey and cook for 2-3 minutes more.

Pour pumpkin into a large crockpot. In a large bowl, stir together milk, wine, and chicken broth. Add brown sugar and orange juice. Stir in onion-turkey mixture, white pepper and pasta sprinkle. Blend into pumpkin in crockpot and cook on low heat for 3-4 hours, stirring occasionally. Make sure soup does not boil. Garnish with parsley before serving.

Serving tip: *Carve out the inside of a pumpkin and cut the top to form a lid. Use the pumpkin as a tureen. Note: This soup is very rich so serve it in cup-size portions. I also microwave the ginger for 25 seconds to soften the skin for easy peeling and chopping.*

Crab Cheese Ball

Yield: 12 servings

    2   packages (8 ounces each) cream cheese, softened

    8   ounces imitation crab, finely chopped

    1   teaspoon Worcestershire sauc

  $^1/_4$ cups finely chopped celery

    1   scallion, finely chopped

  $^1/_4$ teaspoon garlic salt

  $^1/_3$ cup chopped fresh parsley

Beat cream cheese until smooth. Add crab, Worcestershire sauce, celery, scallion, and garlic salt. Blend all together and shape into a ball. Garnish with parsley and serve with your favorite crackers.

Arrange Cheddar and Swiss cheese, turkey and ham on a tray. Garnish with parsley and cherry tomatoes.

Hot Apple Cider Punch

    1   gallon apple cider

    3   cups cider seasoning mix

    3   apple cinnamon or cranberry apple herb teabags

    6   cinnamon sticks (3-4 inches long)

    1   tablespoon brandy flavoring

    2   tablespoons sugar

Mix the apple cider and cider seasoning mix together. Brew the tea with 3 cups of hot water and 3 teabags. Add the tea, cinnamon sticks, brandy flavoring, and sugar to the apple cider mixture. Heat through. Serve in coffee cups.

Donuts

Yield: 24 donuts

    2   cups cooking oil (preferably peanut oil)

    3   cans (8 biscuits per can) prepared biscuits

    2   cups powdered sugar

Heat oil in a 5-quart pan on medium high heat. Poke a hole in the middle of each biscuit. Fry the donuts, turning them over to brown on both sides, for 2-3 minutes. They will puff up while frying. Remove donuts with tongs or slotted spoon. Drain on paper towels. In a small paper bag put powdered sugar. Place warm donuts a few at a time into the bag and shake them to coat with sugar. Place donuts into basket lined with a napkin.

Note: *It is best to make these donuts the day of the party just before serving.*

Fall Memories

Supplies needed:

      Photo of trees turning color.

      Bushel basket filled with fall leaves.

      Rake.

      Pumpkin.

      Indian corn.

      Apple cider.

Discussion questions:

      Pass around the photo. Isn't this a beautiful scene?

Pass around bushel basket with leaves. Do you remember playing in leaf piles when you were a child? Who liked the sound of leaves scrunching under your feet? Have residents scrunch leaves with hands. Show the rake; pass around and have them feel the prongs. How would you use this? Do you remember raking the yard? Pass around and have them feel the pumpkin. Did you carve pumpkins at Halloween? What did you do with the seeds? What would you do with the Indian corn? Have them feel the corn and husk.

Serve fresh apple cider and sing and play the song "When Autumn Leaves Start to Fall" and "I Love Paris."

Leaf Scrapbook

My experience with my aunt taught me the importance of color to Alzheimer's patients. I made a scrapbook of leaves to use in conversation with patients. I picked leaves and copied each leaf on a color copier. You can find pictures of autumn leaves on pages 250-261.

I used this in conversation with individual residents. They can follow one-step directions. With a lower-functioning resident, I would choose a page and ask him to count the stems on the page. Some may be able to identify the colors. Ask questions, such as which leaf is larger? How many leaves are on this page? Can you find the bright red leaves on this page? Which leaf is missing a stem? You can add your own questions as you go.

Note: *Some may even know the names of the leaves, especially the Maple leaf. I actually picked leaves and went to a local print shop and placed the leaves on a color copy machine to reproduce the leaves for my booklet. You can do the same. This project is easy to put together.*

A Booklet of Leaves to Show Changes in Color, Sizes, and Shapes.

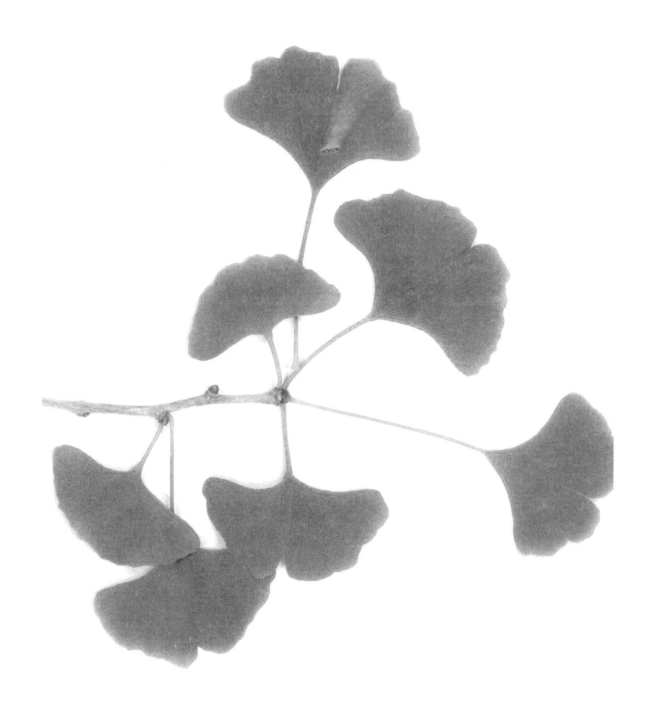

Leaves from a Ginkgo tree.

Note: I have given you a start. You can add many more samples of your own.

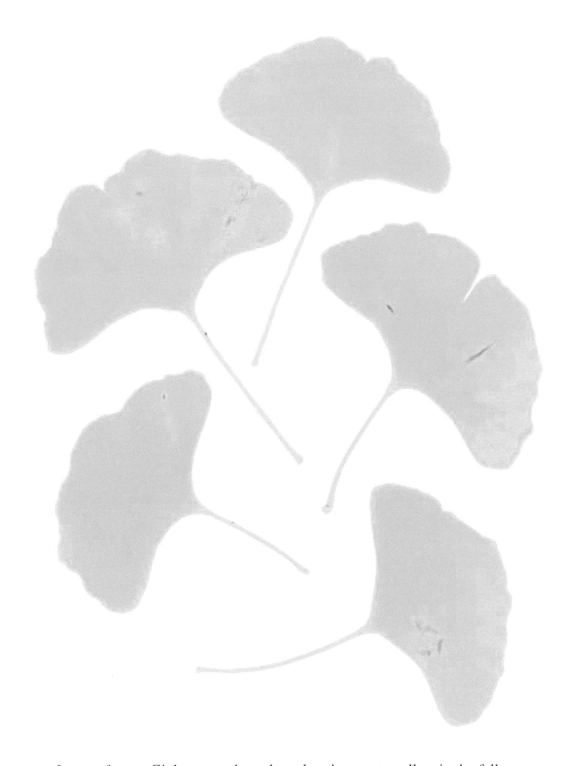

Leaves from a Ginkgo tree show the color changes to yellow in the fall.

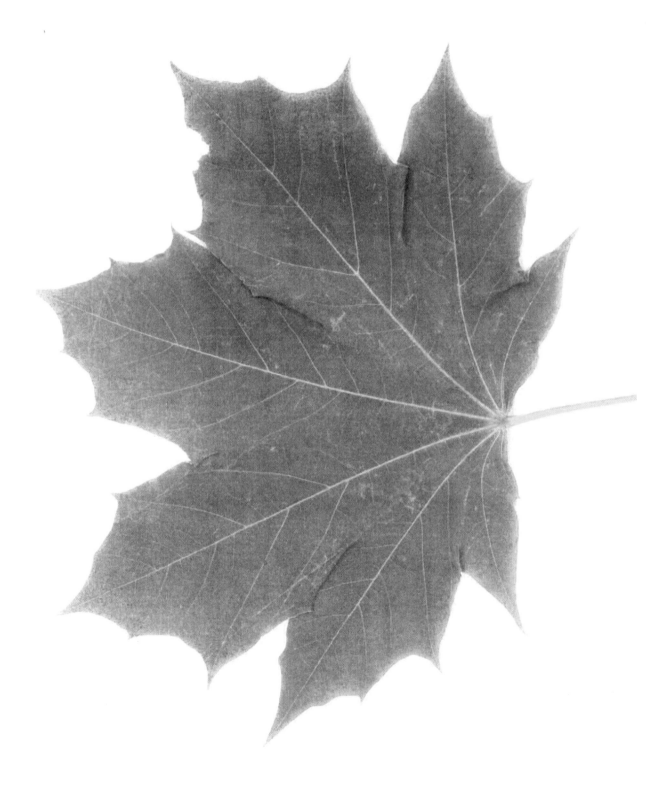

Maple leaf.

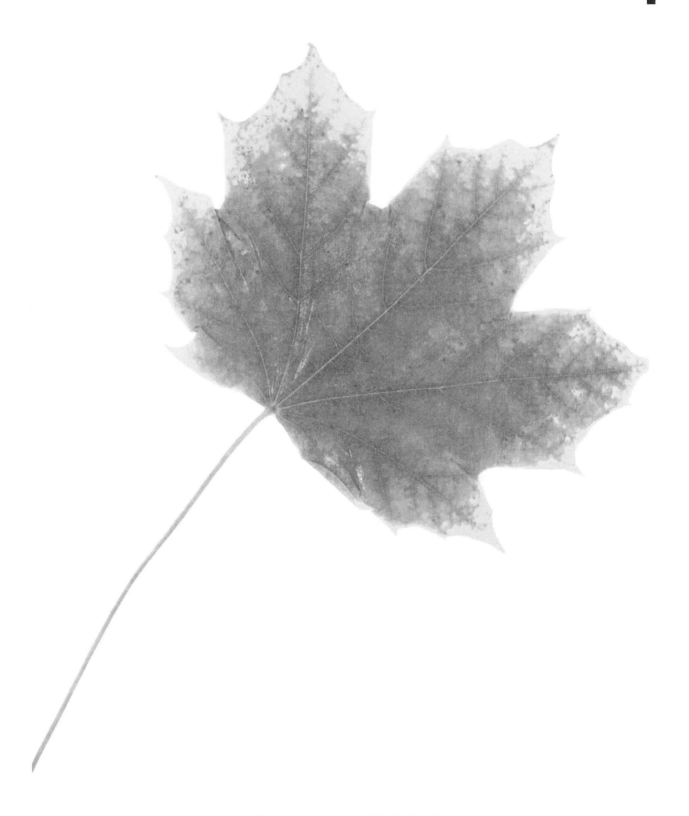

Color change of a Maple leaf.

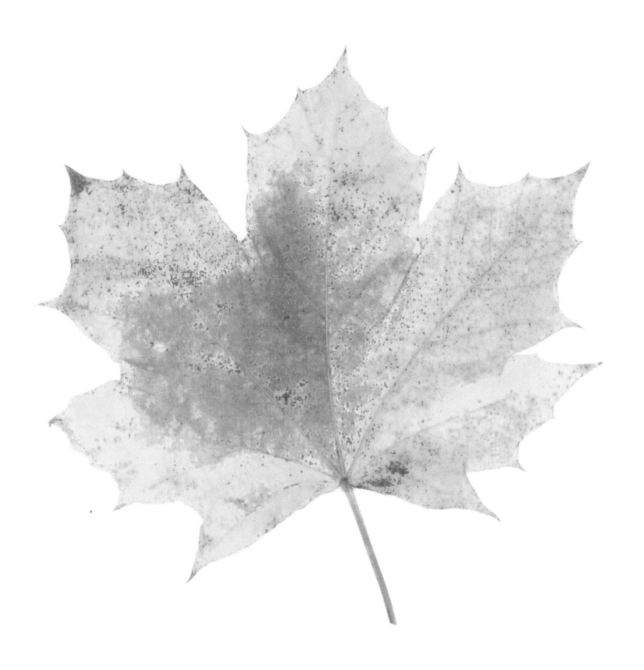

Color change of a Maple leaf.

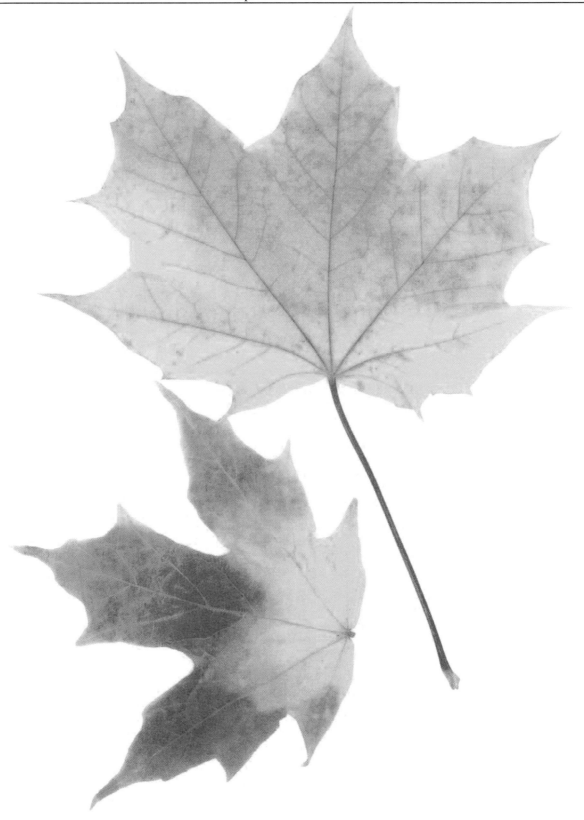

Crimson Maple leaf color change.

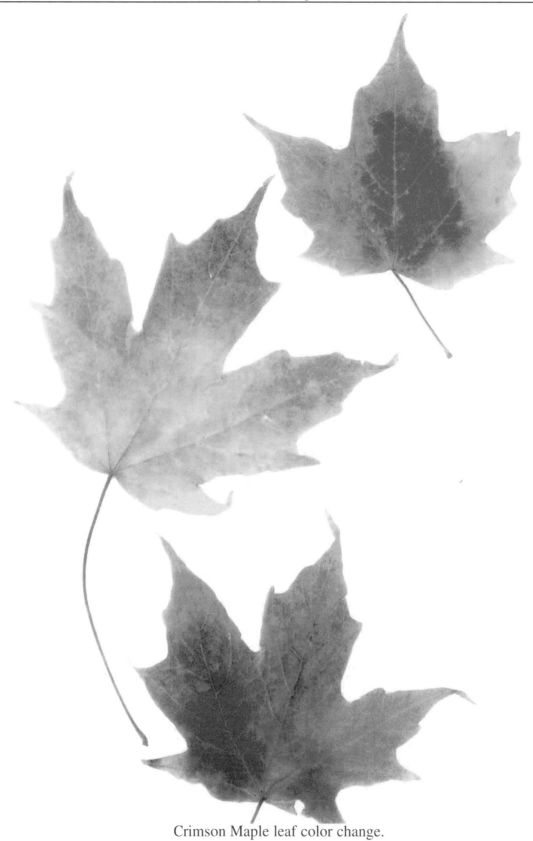

Crimson Maple leaf color change.

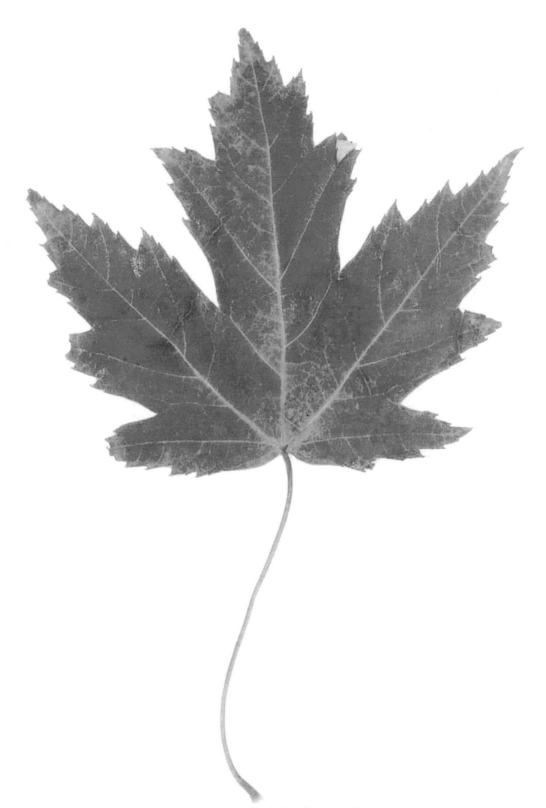

Crimson Maple leaf color change.

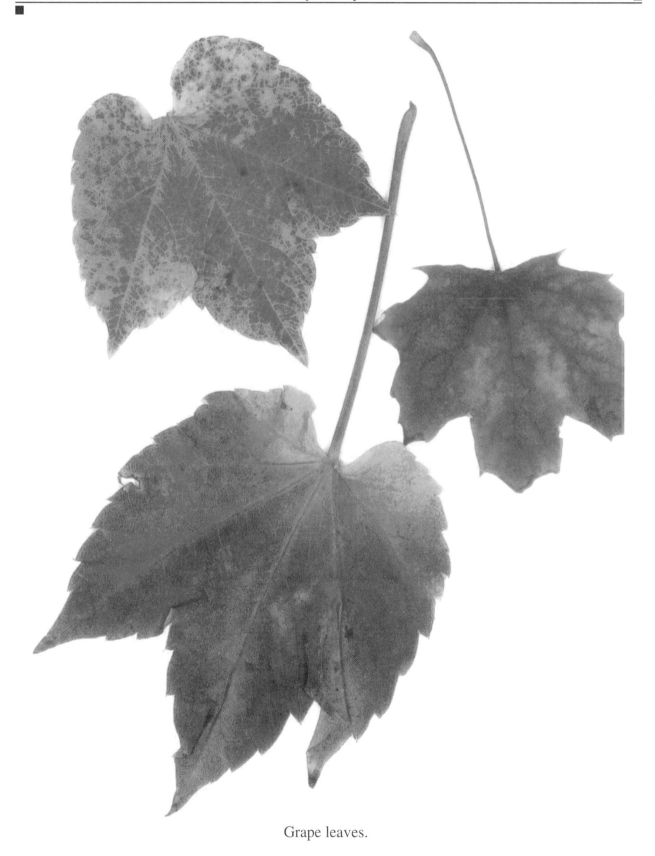

Grape leaves.

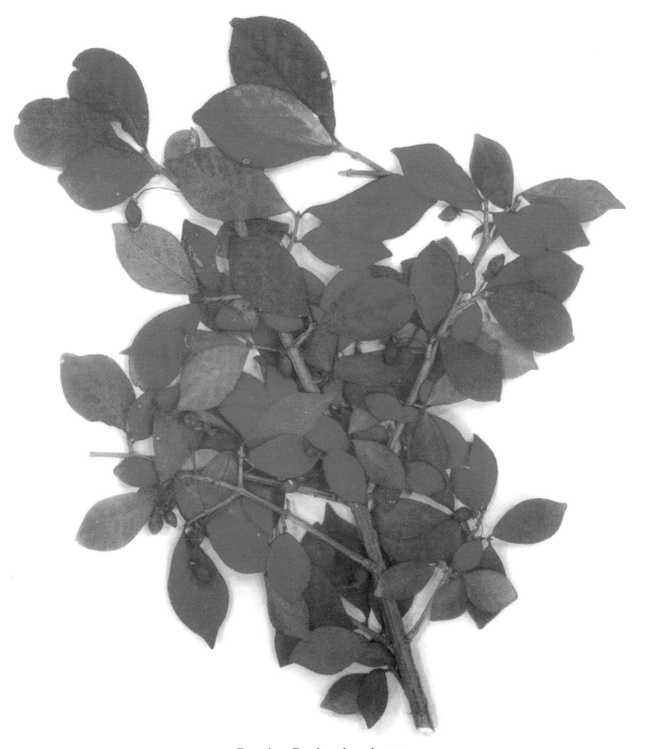

Burning Bush color change.

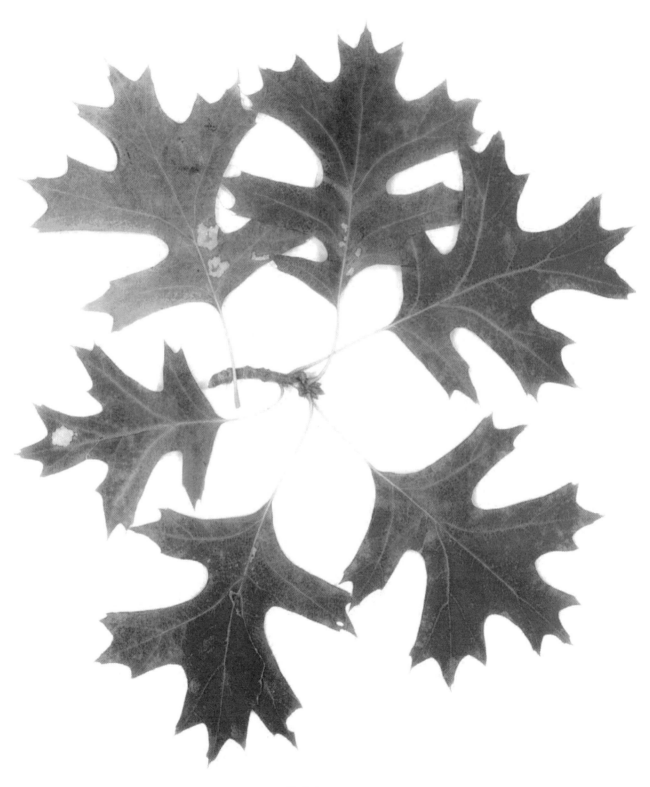

Oak leaves.

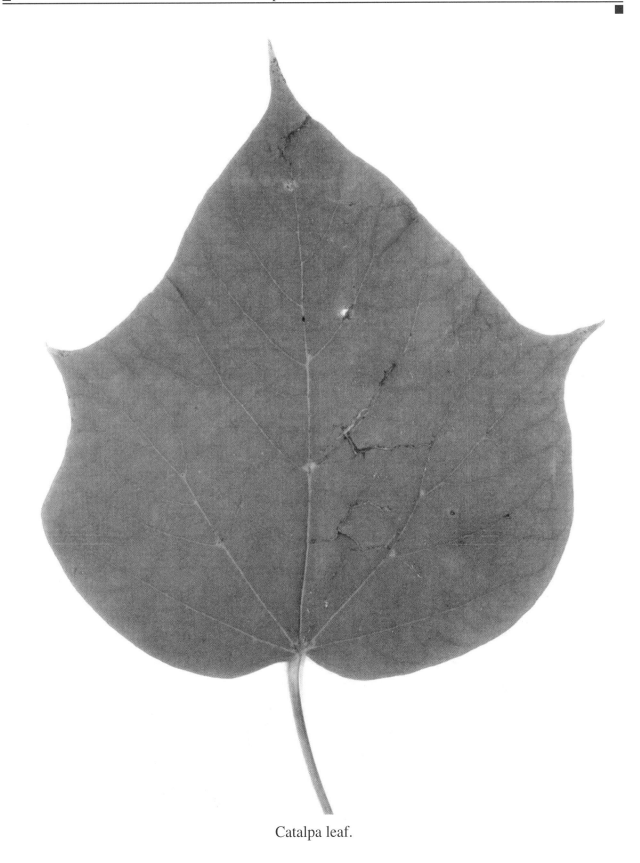

Catalpa leaf.

Chapter 19:

NOVEMBER

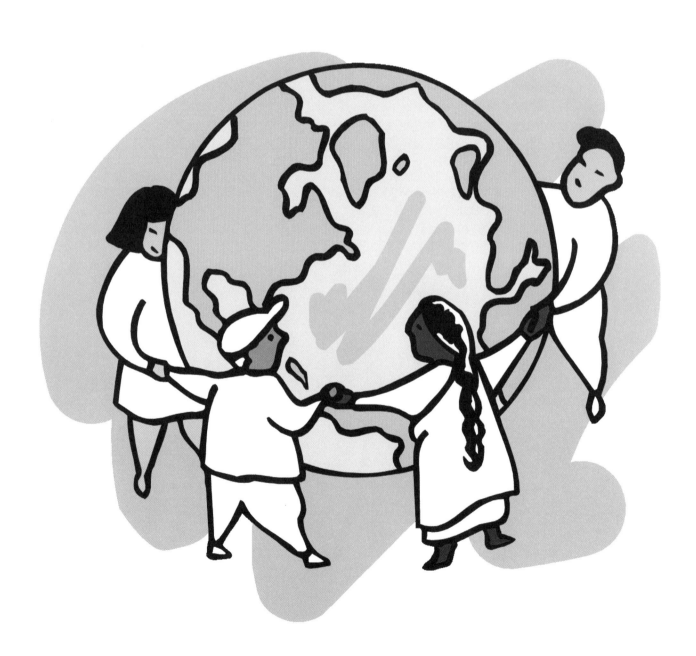

Inspiration: The Meaning of Prayer to the Elderly

I was hired to work with Christian (mostly Catholic) residents, as this is my own background. It's important for any caregiver to learn of the religious beliefs of each person they're caring for, and to help them meet their own religious needs. Many elderly people have strong religious beliefs and rely on daily prayer to comfort them.

Even some Alzheimer's patients and early-stage memory-impaired people are aware that they will die. My mom called out for my dad in her last few days of life. A resident I work with weekly calls out asking for her husband and repeatedly says that she will die. Prayer and religious hymns have a very calming effect on many residents. Many of the elderly recall hymns that they were raised with in their church. They can recall tunes even if they do not remember all the lyrics. Worship services are very meaningful to them. Watching them connect with God is a moving experience.

Inspiration: Rosary and Psalm

The rosary is the prayer that is said by those who practice the Catholic faith. Over the years, many residents I've worked with have requested help with the rosary, so I've gone through the steps here. The rosary is repetitious as it draws people to contemplate on the mysteries of salvation. Catholics begin by saying the Apostle's Creed, followed by the Lord's Prayer and three Hail Marys, one Glory to the Father, followed by one of the mysteries for the given day. The Our Father is then recited.

There are five decades of Hail Marys. It is a tradition to pray the five decades of one of the mysteries of the rosary. The joyful mysteries are used on Mondays and Thursdays and on the Sundays of Advent. The sorrowful mysteries are used on Tuesdays and Fridays and on the Sundays of Lent. The glorious mysteries are used on Wednesdays and Saturdays and on the remaining Sundays of the year.

Apostle's Creed

I believe in God, the Father almighty, creator of heaven and earth.

I believe in Jesus Christ, His only Son, our Lord.

He was conceived by the power of the Holy Spirit and born of the Virgin Mary.

He suffered under Pontius Pilate, was crucified, died and was buried.

He descended to the dead.

On the third day He rose again and is seated at the right hand of the Father.

He will come again to judge the living and the dead.

I believe in the Holy Spirit, the holy Catholic Church, the communion of saints,

the forgiveness of sin, the resurrection of the body, and the life everlasting,

Glory to the Father

Glory to the Father, and to the Son, and to the Holy Spirit;

As it was in the beginning, is now,

And will be for ever.

Amen.

The Lord's Prayer is said before each mystery and after the Apostle's Creed (a total of six times during the reciting of the rosary).

The Lord's Prayer

Our Father Who art in Heaven

Hallowed be thy name

Thy Kingdom come

Thy will be done on earth as it is in heaven.

Give us our daily bread and forgive those who have trespassed against us

And lead us not into temptation, but deliver us from evil. Amen.

The Rosary Can be Concluded With the Following Prayer

Plan A

Hail, holy Queen, mother of mercy,

Hail, our life, our sweetness, and our hopes,

To you we cry, the children of Eve,

To you we send up our sighs, mourning, and weeping in this land of exile,

Turn, then, most gracious advocate, your eyes of mercy toward us;

Lead us home at last and show us the blessed fruit of your womb, Jesus:

O clement, loving, O sweet Virgin Mary.

Plan B

Mary, mother whom we bless, full of grace and tenderness, defend me from the devil's power and greet me in my dying hour.

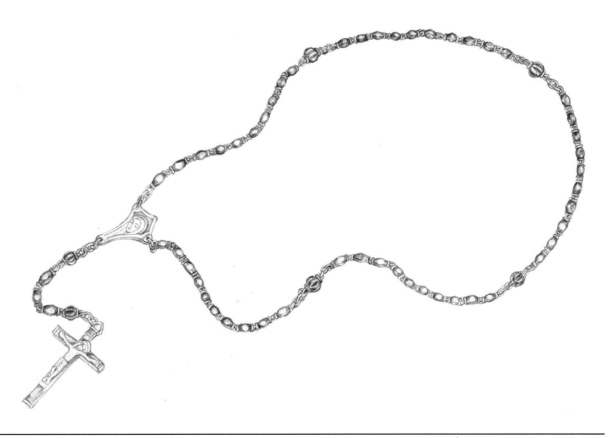

The Joyful Mysteries

1. The Annunciation.

2.The Visitation.

3. The Nativity.

4. The Presentation.

5. The Finding of Jesus in the Temple.

The Sorrowful Mysteries

1. The Agony in the Garden.

2. The Scourging at the Pillar.

3. The Crowning with Thorns.

4. The Carrying of the Cross.

5. The Crucifixion.

The Glorious Mysteries

1. The Resurrection.

2. The Ascension.

3. The Coming of the Holy Spirit.

4. The Assumption of Mary.

5. The Coronation of Mary.

Some of the people say this saying after every decade of the rosary: "Forgive us for our sins. Save us from the fire of Hell. Especially for those in most need of our mercy."

As I worked with the elderly I saw many rosaries on nightstands or around the elderly person's neck. The rosary is a rote verse that many Alzheimer's patients can mimic due to its repetition. I remember saying the rosary with the dying, including my mother. Even though she had Alzheimer's she still could follow me as I said those prayers. By the beginning of the fourth stage she could not say the rosary alone, but she could mimic me as I said the Hail Mary's. My mother said a rosary before she went to bed almost her entire life. She held my hand tight during her last few weeks of her life. I felt a calming effect and a sense of peace as we prayed the rosary.

Hail Mary

Hail Mary, full of grace, the Lord is with you!

Blessed are you among women, and blessed is the fruit of thy womb, Jesus.

Holy Mary, Mother of God, pray for us sinners, now and at the hour of our death.

Amen.

Many facilities have the rosary as an activity. If you are not comfortable saying the rosary ask a volunteer to come in and recite the rosary. Make a special time of the week or month for this activity. At one of the facilities where I worked, a 102-year-old woman led the rosary for the small group. She did an excellent job.

I also own both Catholic and Protestant Bibles and carried them with me for one-on-one visits.

I always asked if it was okay to read the Bible. I would find out the residents' favorite verses as I got to know them.

Psalm 100 is a song of praise and a morning prayer. Most older Christians know this psalm.

> Sing joyfully to the Lord, all you lands;
> Serve the Lord with gladness;
> Come before Him with joyful song.
> Know that the Lord is God;
> He made us, we are His people, the flock He tends.
> Enter His gates with thanksgiving, His courts with praise;
> Give thanks to him; bless his name, for He is good;
> The Lord, whose kindness endures forever, and His faithfulness, to all
> generations.

Psalm 13 is a Plea in Difficult Times.

Out of the depths I cry to You, O Lord;
Lord, hear my voice!
Let Your ears be attentive to my voice in supplication;
If you, O Lord, mark iniquities, Lord, who can stand?
But with You is forgiveness, that You may be revered.
I trust in the Lord;
My soul trusts in his word.
My soul waits for the Lord more than sentinels wait for the dawn.
More than sentinels wait for the dawn, let Israel wait for the Lord.
For with the Lord is kindness and with Him is plenteous redemption;
And He will redeem Israel from all their iniquities.

Psalm 150 The Hymn of Praise

Praise the Lord in his sanctuary,
Praise Him in the firmament of his strength.
Praise Him for his mighty deeds,
Praise Him for his sovereign majesty.
Praise Him with the blast of the trumpet,
Praise Him with lyre and harp,
Praise Him with timbrel and dance,
Praise Him with strings and pipe,
Praise Him with sounding cymbals.
Let everything that has breath
Praise the Lord! Alleluia.

Note: *Each week, invite a different religious leader to come in and have a service. Also have hymns for the residents to sing. They appreciate this time.*

Inspiration: Poetry, Reflections, and Favorite Hymns

I often read poems from *Favorite Poems Old and New* selected by Helen Ferris (copyright 1957, first edition). This book is very old but I have found it appeals to the Alzheimer's patients. It is a good tool to describe simple things like the seasons and trees, and it makes them feel good. Many times I would walk around the facility and read one-to-one from this book. Each poem is relatively short. The descriptions are outstanding and easy to understand.

I enjoyed reading to a resident who had been a librarian in a facility where I worked. I still see her smiling face and bright eyes as I write this. She didn't like to participate in activities much, but she could sit for a half hour and listen to poetry. She is now in heaven.

Kindness

Kindness comes from a place in the heart. A few words of care, a smile, a handful of hope…these are little things but too important to leave in words unsaid, or deed undone. Simple kindnesses are like shared joys: nurture the seed and a flower will grow. So give what you have to someone…. It may mean more than you'll ever know.

Each time you give a kindness away, it's a gift you'll be giving to yourself.

—Author unknown

Look busy! Jesus is coming!

(Bumper sticker)

"Just living", said the butterfly, "is not enough.

You must have sunshine, freedom, and a little flower."

—Hans Christian Anderson

Love

Love is everything. It is making of dreams and of promises to keep.

It is having stars in your eyes and tomorrows in your heart.

It is the giving of songs and of silences and the holding of memories only the heart can see.

Love can be the sudden magic of a moment or as subtle as a glance from across a room. It can be felt in the soft squeezing of hands, a gentle hug from a child, or the sharing of whispers only two hearts can hear.

Without love in our hearts, our lives would be as empty as a tomorrow without a dream.

—Author unknown

I Said a Prayer for You Today

I said a prayer for you today and know God must have heard

I felt the answer in my heart

Although He spoke no word!

I didn't ask for wealth or fame

(I knew you wouldn't mind)

I asked Him to send treasures

Of a far more lasting kind!

I asked that He'd be near you

At the start of each day

To grant you health and blessings

And friends to share your way!

I asked for happiness for you

In all things great and small

But it was for His loving care

I prayed the most of all.

—Author unknown

My Prayer

To love we must accept ourselves.

Lord, help me see each present moment as my opportunity to:

Recognize Your act of eternal creation;

Find Your goodness in myself and others;

and may my love always grow.

—Stephen Nekola

Favorite Hymns

"Jesus Loves Me"

"The Old 100th Psalm"

"Now Thank We All Our God"

"Bringing in the Sheaves"

"In the Garden"

"Thou Almighty King"

"God of Our Fathers"

"Ave Maria"

"Rock of Ages"

"Swing Low, Sweet Chariot"

"We Shall Overcome"

"We Gather Together"

"Sweet By and By"

"Praise God From Whom All Blessings Flow"

"Onward Christian Soldiers"

"The Old Rugged Cross"

"O Come O Come Emmanuel"

"Blest Be the Tie That Binds"

"Blessed Assurance"

"The Church in the Wildwood"

"Give Me That Old Time Religion"

"I Love to Tell the Story"

"Joshua Fit de Battle of Jericho"

"Praise to the Lord, the Almighty"

"Prayer of Thanksgiving"

"Stand Up! Stand Up! for Jesus"

"What a Friend We Have in Jesus"

"Whispering Hope"

"Amazing Grace"

I find that the omichord (an instrument similar to an autoharp) is great for singing the hymns. It is a softer instrument and the residents can hum along the tune. They can hear the chords on this instrument. A few may know a couple of the words or lines in different songs. Many elderly people grew up with the hymn music and will enjoy every minute of these songs.

Reminiscing

While I was waiting for the activity director to come to lead me to the activity room, one of the residents of the independent living facility was sitting in the front waiting room. I greeted her, and she began to talk to me about her younger years. She said she had lived on Third Street in Milwaukee many years before. She'd had a purebred dog as a young girl that was quite unusual. Her mother would tie a note on a basket and put the basket around this large dog's neck. He would go to the grocery store for her mother. Her mom would let the grocery lady know that her dog was on the way. The dog would scratch at the door and wait for the lady to come fetch the basket and grocery list. He sat on the step waiting for the order to be filled. The grocery lady would put the bill into the basket and the basket around the dog's neck. Many times her mother ordered hot dogs and the dog did not even eat the hot dogs or one morsel of food. He simply got the groceries back safely to their home. I thought that was quite a story.

Spice of Life

This exercise helps the Alzheimer's resident to recall good foods made with each spice. I did this exercise with the lower-functioning Alzheimer's patients. It was well received. The residents participated fairly well and responded to the smells of the various spices.

Spices and Their Uses

Chinese five-spice (stir fry).
Barbecue spice (chicken for a cookout).
Bay leaves (soups).
Seafood spice (fish).
Chili powder (chili).
Cayenne pepper (spicy hot chili).
Garlic herb seasoning (chicken).
Cloves (pumpkin pie and general baking).
Italian seasoning (spaghetti and lasagna).
Lemon pepper (chicken or fish).
Parsley flakes (parsleyed potatoes and garnishes for salads).
Cumin (Mexican foods).
Dill weed (Greek food).
Chives (sour cream for baked potatoes).
Cinnamon (coffee cakes and cookies).

For this activity, I wore a chef's hat and a chef's coat to get the folks thinking "food." They knew I was a chef. One woman who had been the head cook at a high school asked if she could wear my hat. I put it on her and asked what her favorite food was that she'd prepared for the students. She said, "Oh, strudel! There was never enough. We don't get strudel here either."

She went on, "A good cook never measures—she just knows. She puts the spices into her hand and can tell how much to add."

With help we passed the spices around one by one and talked about the name of the spice and how it is used in various foods and dishes. The residents really reacted in a positive manner when we talked about cloves in pumpkin pie. We reminisced about Thanksgiving Day, and I told them a story about my neighbor. Her husband had to wear special cotton socks that only came in white, so she used to dye them black, and she used her big turkey roaster to do it in. When she used her roaster on Thanksgiving Day one year, she forgot to wipe out the pan before she roasted her turkey—and the turkey turned black from the dye! That Thanksgiving she served baked chicken, and she never used the roaster to dye socks again.

One woman kept saying that she wanted to go. I got her to stay in the group by telling her I had come especially to see her and would be disappointed if she left. She mentioned leaving several times, but she stayed. I said, "You need to have some patience." "I know, I know," she replied. "Patience is a virtue, and I have none."

A Look at the World

At the beginning of the program, heat apple cider and add cinnamon sticks. Let the smell permeate the room.

I started with exercise, tossing an inflated plastic globe. The residents enjoyed looking at the map of the world. After exercising, play live music.

Songs with world as part of the title or in the lyrics of the song:
"Let the Rest of the World Go By"
"He's Got the Whole World in His Hands"
"Around the World in Eighty Days"
"If You Were the Only Girl in the World"
"What the World Needs Now"
"I've Got the World on a String"
"We Are the World"

"This Is My Father's World"
"The Most Beautiful Girl in the World"
"Small World"
"The World Is Waiting for the Sunrise"
"Wonderful, Wonderful"
"It's a Marshmallow World"

Patriotic songs
"My Country 'Tis of Thee"
"America the Beautiful"
"God Bless America"

Conclude the program by serving hot cider and coffee.

Planting Paperwhite Bulbs

Supplies needed per container of bulbs:

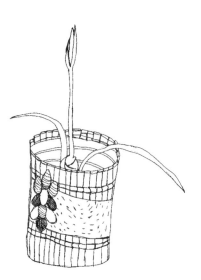

1 can, 6-inches in diameter and 6-inches high (the type of
can cashews come in works well).
1 bag wooden clothespins (100 per bag) with long springs
(One bag should cover 2 cashew nut cans. However, there
will not be enough if any of the clothespins are broken
or bent. I recommend buying 1 bag for every 2 projects,
plus 1 extra).
Hot-glue gun.
$3/4$ yard $2^1/_2$ to 3-inch wide ribbon.
3 pieces wagon wheel pasta.
Small, clean rocks to fill the can (you can purchase land-
scaping rocks from a garden center).
3 paperwhite bulbs.
Water.

Clean the cans, removing the labels. Help residents pull the clothespins apart and save the springs for hanging plants. A volunteer can hot-glue the flat side of each clothespin to the can with the thin part of the clothespin at the bottom of the can. Make sure one clothespin touches the other side by side. It takes 25 whole clothespins per row or a total of 50 per can. Repeat the second row, butting the thicker part with the first row of clothespins.

Note: Closely supervise the use of the hot-glue gun, as the glue can burn skin. You can sit with the residents and use white glue instead to glue on the clothespins if you have the time. It is a good exercise for you and the residents to share time together. It makes the residents feel good when they can help.

Hot-glue the ribbon around the middle of the can. Hot-glue wagon wheel pasta to form flower petals on the front of the can. (You can use pasta seashells instead, or any shapes you desire.)

Fill the can with small rocks to about 1 inch from the top. Cover rocks with cold water. Place three paperwhite bulbs on top of the rocks in each can, with the stem side up and root down. Make sure the water is touching the root. Watch the paperwhites grow. Keep the plants watered. The residents enjoy watering and seeing the paperwhites grow.

A Thanksgiving Friendship Coffee Hour

Relax and enjoy having a cup of coffee and reminiscing about friendships, making everyone feel like a part of the group.

Supplies needed:
Decaffeinated coffee beans or ground coffee in a variety of flavors.
I brought:
Highlander Grogg (a mixture of hazelnut, caramel, and cinnamon).

Raspberry cream.	Apricot cream.
Cinnamon.	Cranberry.
Chocolate mint.	Hazelnut.
Almond.	Coconut cream.

1 sugar dipper* per person.
  (*stirring stick with crystallized sugar at the end. The sugar
  dissolves when stirred into coffee or tea. Available at coffee stores.)
1 small bowl or cup per coffee flavor.
Coffeepot.
Coffee cups.
Cream and sugar.

The smell is wonderful. Each coffee was stored in a separate bag. I made sure the bags were airtight to ensure the freshness of the flavors. I selected the above coffees because each aroma is distinctive. I placed each type of beans into a cup and labeled it. I passed the cups around so that the residents could smell the beans. While this activity was taking place Highlander Grogg coffee was brewing and the scent permeated the room.

A gentleman that was in the fourth stage of Alzheimer's in a geri chair was down for the session. I had him smell the chocolate mint coffee beans. He raised his eyebrows and opened his eyes somewhat. That was a very neat encounter.

The coconut cream and almond are strong smells that help the resident's olfactory stimuli. It was fun watching the residents' delightful facial expressions as they smelled each flavored coffee. We served residents that wanted to taste the brewed coffee. As they were drinking their coffee we read sayings and talked about the meaning of sharing a cup of coffee with a friend. I had a coffee mug with a heart and house on the mug. It read, "Welcome friends." I passed it around to the residents so that they could hold the big handle on the cup. I also passed around an extra large cup and said a person could have one big cup of coffee and lots of conversation with a friend. I passed a card around with a picture of a teacup. It read "Thinking of you warms my heart." (See page 277)

A Friend

I have a friend in high places
who lives within the hearts of people.
When I speak to people, I speak to my friend
And my friend always answers

—From a print by Sally Huss. Author unknown.

One lady named her husband as her best friend. She missed him so. She stated, "I guess he is at home now."

An activity person said, "No, your husband is dead."

She responded, "No he is not; he is at home."

I then said, "Yes, indeed, he is in a higher place, in a heavenly home looking down at you today." She accepted that answer from me and smiled.

I make my own cards, and some of my favorite sayings for them are:

The best and most beautiful gifts cannot be seen or even
   touched they must be felt with the heart.
Sow courtesy and reap friendship.
Plant kindness and gather love.
Thank you for being a special friend.
Friends are like flowers that never fade.
You make me happy because you are my dear friend.
What are friends for?
You pick your friends but not your family.
Friendship is like a sweet bouquet of hearts.
That is where love and kindness starts.
Friendship comes from the heart.
A millionaire cannot buy friendship!

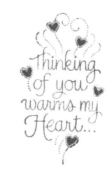

The cards were passed around to the residents. They enjoyed the colors of the cards and the sayings. Most of the group expressed the value of friendship. It was not something that money could buy. There were a couple of people that had made friends in the group. A good friend, like an old quilt, is both a treasure and a comfort.

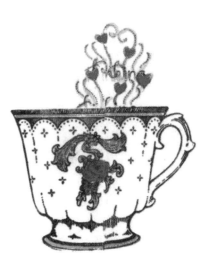

I played songs to express the value of friendship:
   "Jesus Loves Me"
   "Moonlight Bay"
   "Meet Me in Dreamland"
   "Down by the Old Mill Stream"
   "Shine on Harvest Moon"
   "Sewanee"
   "They Didn't Believe Me"
   "Too-Ra-Loo-Ra-Loo-Ra"
   (A lullaby to remind them of being a friend to a baby or small child.)
   "You Made Me Love You"
   "My Jesus I Love Thee"
   "A Beautiful Friendship"
   "Got a Date With an Angel"

"Joyful, Joyful, We Adore Thee" (Ode to Joy)
"I Love to Tell the Story"
"Red Sails in the Sunset"
"Sugartime"
"Joshua Fit de Battle of Jericho"

We concluded the program with the song "Joshua Fit de Battle of Jericho," getting some of the residents to clap and use the rhythmic instruments.

Thanksgiving

I dressed up like a pilgrim. I showed off my costume to the residents to explain how the pilgrims looked in the 1600s. I also showed pictures of pilgrim children. The residents enjoyed seeing the fashions of that time. One lady enjoyed wearing my hat. I set up the table with a horn of plenty filled with mini pumpkins, leaves, gourds, and a variety of squash. I had scented candles shaped like pilgrim children that I passed around to the residents. They could smell the candles and see how the child figures looked. They also could feel the waxy texture. I also passed vegetables for the residents to see and touch. A large stuffed turkey sat in the middle of the table with various colored feathers. We made turkey art sculptures and baked a pumpkin pie to give great aroma in the activity room. I then told a story about Thanksgiving and concluded the program with a poem and a song.

Pumpkin Pie

Pie crust (single crust):

1$^1/_2$	cups flour
$^1/_2$	teaspoon sugar
$^1/_2$	teaspoon salt
$^3/_4$	cup shortening
1	beaten egg
2-3	tablespoons ice water
1	teaspoon vinegar

Preheat oven to 425 degrees. In a medium bowl, mix flour, sugar, and salt. Cut in shortening until pea-sized crumbs form. Add the beaten egg to 2 tablespoons ice water along with the vinegar. Blend well, add to flour mixture and blend until dough just holds together, adding more ice water if necessary. Roll out dough between two pieces of waxed paper to 1-inch larger than inverted pie pan. Peel off top piece of waxed paper. Place dough in pie pan; remove remaining waxed paper. Tuck edges of dough under to form a border even with edges of pan. Flute crust. Cover edges with $1^1/_2$-inch-wide strip of foil. Set aside.

Following directions on the pumpkin pie can, mix up the pumpkin pie filling. Ingredients needed are as following:

> 1 can (16 ounces) pumpkin pie filling
> Granulated sugar
> Salt
> Ground cloves
> Ground ginger
> Ground cinnamon
> Eggs
> Evaporated milk

Pour filling in the piecrust. Bake for 15 minutes. Reduce temperature to 350 degrees. Bake 40-50 minutes more or until knife inserted in the middle of the pie filling comes out clean. Cool and refrigerate. Serve with whipped topping.

Turkey Food Art Project

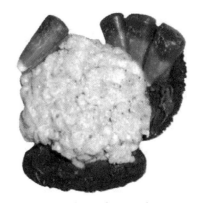

Supplies needed:

3 T	Margarine.
8 cups	Rice Krispies cereal.
4 cups	miniature marshmallows.
25	Oreo sandwich cookies.
100	Brown and orange colored candy corn.
1	16 oz. can prepared milk chocolate frosting.

Follow instructions on the cereal box to make Rice Krispie treats. Form the mixture into $2^1/_2$- to 3-inch balls. Place one candy corn in the middle of each ball for the beak. Use the chocolate frosting like a glue. Take an Oreo apart. Set the ball on a frosted cookie half to use as a stand. Use the frosting like glue to press the other half of the of the Oreo onto the back of the ball to represent the tail of the turkey. For tail feathers, stick three candy corn between the ball and the cookie tail with frosting. Make these treats for families and visitors or use as gifts for a Thanksgiving gathering. Yield: 25 turkeys.

Story: How Thanksgiving First Began

Thanksgiving began with the pilgrims. King James I did not allow religious freedom in England. A group decided to leave their homeland and journey to America. They became known as the Separatists. William Bradford named these folks the pilgrims. Of the 102 passengers, there were only 42 Separatists and the remainder just wanted to come to America to start a new life. Fifteen of the passengers were children. Fifteen of the male passengers were named John and five of the females were named Mary. That had to be confusing to have so many Johns and Marys on board especially since they all wore the same style hats. They packed plenty of salt beef, cheese, biscuits, onions, dried peas, and beans for the long journey across the deep waters. They boarded the *Mayflower* in August 1620 and left Plymouth, England. They were heading for the Hudson River, for the area known as New York City today.

Now, mind you, the *Mayflower* was only 90 feet long and 25 feet wide—the size of two school buses. Depending on the weather, they could go no more than two miles an hour, or 48 miles a day. Can you imagine 102 passengers plus 20 sailors on such a small ship? There were no bathroom facilities, nor beds to sleep in, nor a kitchen to heat food. The pilgrims learned to pray, play, and work together on the trip. They ate all food cold. A joy came when a baby was born on the *Mayflower*. The baby boy was name Oceanus. At one point they turned back to England. It was not until their second attempt that they landed at Plymouth, Massachusetts, after 66 days on the voyage from Plymouth, England. Many were cold, seasick, and homesick. Some had died on the way. Nevertheless, the pilgrims gave thanks to God for a safe voyage. They held a dream in their hearts of arriving in America safely.

The pilgrims built their homes at Plymouth. In 1621 when spring came, the snow melted and the pilgrims built barns. However, winter brought bitter cold. The pilgrims had very little to eat. They met friendly Indians who helped them learn how to work the land and survive in America.

Samoset could speak English because he had learned the language from fishermen from Maine. Squanto was an exceptionally good friend. He was the last Indian from the Pawtucket tribe. His people had all died of smallpox. He taught the pilgrims how to plant wheat, beans, potatoes, spinach, squash, and pumpkins. Squanto and Samoset also taught the pilgrims how to hunt and fish. The pilgrims learned to trap rabbits and turkey and how to hunt deer and bear. By the following winter the pilgrims could fill their barns with food. They had plenty to eat for the entire winter.

The pilgrims invited their Indian friends to celebrate. Much to the pilgrims' surprise, 91 Indians showed up for the feast. They feasted for three days on fish, turkey, corn, beans, pumpkins, and squash. Without the Indians' help, the pilgrims would have not survived to celebrate Thanksgiving. The pilgrims continued to live peacefully with the Wampanoag Indian tribe as they helped each other for the next 55 years.

In 1789 George Washington (our first president of the United States) declared Thanksgiving a national holiday. Today we celebrate Thanksgiving each year on the fourth Thursday of November. Canada celebrates Thanksgiving in October. Other countries have harvest celebrations during other months of the year in spring and fall. Now as Americans we have the freedom to celebrate Thanksgiving with our families and friends, feasting on our favorite Thanksgiving foods.

Thanksgiving Questions for Discussion:

■ Would you believe that Americans consume almost 45 million turkeys at Thanksgiving?

■ Did you know that Ben Franklin wanted to declare the turkey a national bird? Congress voted his suggestion down and the bald eagle became the national bird instead.

■ Do you know why the turkey did not eat much on Thanksgiving day? He was stuffed!

To conclude the program, form a circle and join hands and recite the poem "We Thank Thee" (*Favorite Poems, Old and New*, by Helen Ferris). Play and sing, "Now Thank We All Our God."

Chapter 20:

DECEMBER

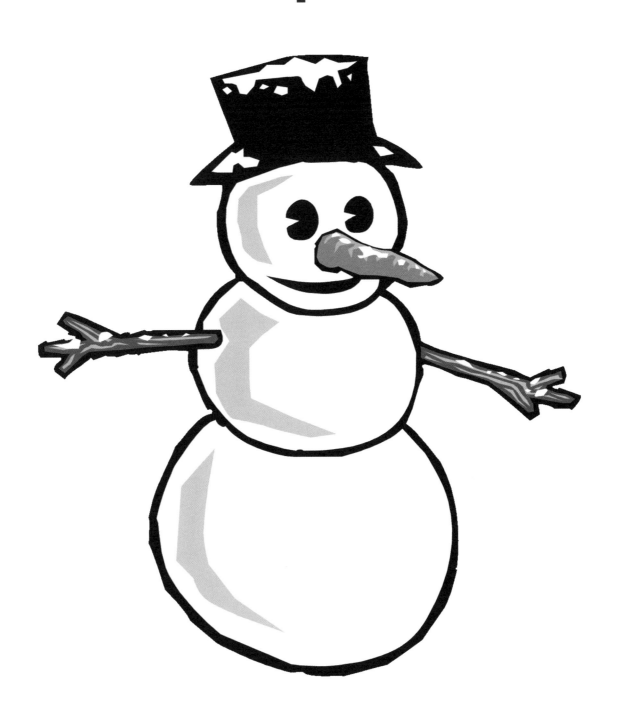

Sorting Socks and Other Items

This activity can be done year-round with a variety of socks. During the holiday season, I brought socks with Christmas patterns. Sorting socks is something most people have done all their lives. I make a pile of all the socks and work with one or two people to help them pick out the colors and the figures on the socks to match the pairs together. For variety, I sometimes have them fold towels and napkins.

I also have different types of pastas and nuts for the residents to sort. I have a board with pasta shapes glued onto it, and another board with nuts, to use as guides. I use trays or butter containers for sorting. For the men I have nuts, bolts, and nails to sort. I use a toolbox for the sorting of nuts and bolts. Many first- and second-stage Alzheimer's patients don't mind sorting especially if they feel useful.

Sometimes I'd wash off bingo chips and have the residents dry them. They would sort the red from the blue chips. They also can recognize sizes, colors, and shapes.

I took old socks with holes and asked the residents to please find the holes in the socks so we could darn them. They could put a hand in the sock to find the holes and feel the textures such as cotton, wool, or nylon. Many people in a care facility feel lonely, bored, and useless. Keeping them active helps them to feel good about their self-esteem and helps prevent chronic depression.

Reminiscing: Remembering Christmases Past

Supplies needed: Christmas toys and decorations. I brought:

> 2 teddy bears dressed in velvet Christmas outfits (1 female and 1 male).
> 1 December page from a calendar.
> 1 sprig of mistletoe.
> 1 large stuffed, musical Frosty the Snowman.
> 1 snowman made of fleece.
> 1 box wrapped like a present with a big red bow.
> > (I have two toy kittens that pop up from my box and sing
> > Christmas songs.)

1 nativity scene.

1 small Christmas tree.

1 candy cane.

1 silver bell.

1 tablecloth with an outdoor winter scene.

6 Christmas stockings.

> (1 filled with sugar, 1 filled with flour, 1 filled with cinnamon sticks, 1 filled with cloves, 1 filled with oatmeal, 1 filled with coal.)

1 chestnut.

Start out with a big circle around December 25 and the year on the calendar. Count how many days to Christmas. Play the song "The Night Before Christmas" with the residents. Recite the poem "A Visit From St. Nicholas" by Clement Clarke Moore. While I was reading the poem, a resident said each word with me and even completed my sentences. It was what she learned in school years ago. Her long-term memory was still good.

Have a resident put a hand into the stocking with the coal. Play and sing "Frosty The Snowman" and display the snowman. Let them feel and see the snowman. Let the residents feel the velvet clothing and the fur on the bears.

The kitten music box received many favorable comments. One lady watched the kittens sing and watched the box lid open and close in between each song. She was a cat lover and fussed over the kittens. The residents enjoyed the tablecloth with the pictures of kids skating, the horse and carriage, trees, Grandma's farm,. and a sleigh ride with Mom and Dad. It brought back fond memories of the good old days.

Each person can put an ornament with their name on the Christmas tree. Sing "O Christmas Tree." Many residents could remember cutting down a Christmas tree with their family. It was a meaningful family gathering. The residents had many smiles while talking about putting up the tree, baking, and shopping for Christmas.

The candy cane has a story behind it. A candy maker in Indiana wanted to make a candy that would act as a witness, so he made the Christmas candy cane. He incorporated several symbols for the birth, ministry, and death of Jesus Christ. He began with a stick of pure white hard candy, white to symbolize the virgin's birth and the sinless nature of Jesus. Hard symbolized the solid rock, the foundation of the church and the firmness of the promises of God. The candy maker made the candy in the form of a J to represent the precious name of Jesus. It could also represent the staff of the good shepherd which he reaches down into the world to lift out the fallen lambs like all sheep have gone astray. Thinking that the candy was somewhat plain, the candy maker stained it with red stripes. He used three small stripes to show the stripes of the scourging Jesus received by which we are healed. The large red stripes were for the blood shed by Christ on the cross so that we could have a promise of eternal life. Eventually, the candy became known as a candy cane. It is a meaningless decoration seen at Christmas time. The meaning is subtle for those who "have eyes to see and ears to hear." Hopefully this symbol will again be used to witness to the wonder of Jesus and his great love that came down at Christmas and remain the ultimate dominate source in the universe today. Display the candy cane with the red stripe to show the true meaning of Christmas.

For the project I put up the manger and placed Jesus, Mary, and Joseph inside the crib area. Also I displayed the three kings, a drummer boy, a shepherd, a sheep, and an angel. I talked about the words in the following songs to discuss the coming of Christ ("Away in the Manger," "We Three Kings of Orient Are," "The Drummer Boy," "O Little Town of Bethlehem," "Oh Holy Night," "Joy to the World," "Angels From the Realm on High," "Angels We Have Heard on High," "The First Noel," "It Came Upon a Midnight Clear," "While Shepherds Watched the Flocks by Night," "Christ Was Born on Christmas Day," "What Child Is This," and "Silent Night").

Many of the residents could hum the tunes and relate to Christmas through the music. While going through the songs a resident in the group put her hands on the table and began to pretend to play the piano as she hummed and sang many of the words to the songs. She had played piano in her younger days. It was delightful to watch her participate. Others hummed and pointed to the different figures in the manger. Many of the residents' faces lit up with the various Christmas songs.

Baking Christmas cookies and making a ham was a holiday tradition for many female residents. I had residents put their fingers into the socks to feel and smell the sugar, flour, cinnamon sticks, oatmeal, and cloves. One resident said, "Yes, cloves. Use the cloves on ham." She said it was always tradition to have ham at the holidays at her home. Play the song "Christmas Is."

Let the residents feel the hardness of the chestnut shell. Play the song "Merry Christmas to You." Play the song "Silver Bells" as a symbol for the silver bell. End the program with "You're All I Want for Christmas."

Making a Candy Cane Candle

Supplies needed:

Lid from a 12-oz. frozen juice can.
Green or red felt.
Hot glue gun.
Glue stick.
Four 5$\frac{1}{2}$-inch candy canes.
12-inch taper candle.
3 small silk poinsettia flowers.

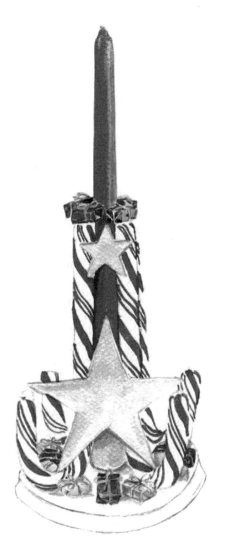

Place the juice lid on the felt and trace a circle. Cut out the circle and glue the felt to the bottom of the can lid. Glue the four candy canes to the candle, placing the hooks curving outward to make the feet of the candle. Hot-glue tiny presents on the top and bottom of the candy canes. Hot glue the stars at the base and on the middle of the candle.

Note: You can use silk poinsettia instead of stars.

Cutout Sugar Cookies

Yield: 3 dozen medium cookies.

$1/2$	cup butter, softened
$1/2$	cup margarine, softened
1	cup sugar
2	eggs
$2^1/_2$-3	cups flour
1	teaspoon baking soda
1	teaspoon nutmeg

Preheat oven to 350 degrees. Cream butter, margarine, and sugar together. Add the eggs and beat well. Add $2^1/_2$ cups flour, baking soda, and nutmeg. Sprinkle some of the extra flour on the board. Dust hands with flour and knead the dough to form a ball. Divide the dough into 3 or 4 small balls. Use floured rolling pin to roll out each ball to $1/8$- to $1/4$-inch thick on floured cutting board. Use floured Christmas cookie cutters to cut out the dough. Place cookies on ungreased cookie sheet and bake 10-15 minutes. Cookies should stay white on top and light golden color on the bottom. Cool and cover with icing, decorate and store in airtight container.

Note: You can use one cup of butter total if you choose not to use margarine.

Cookie Icing

1	teaspoon almond extract
$1/4$	teaspoon salt
$1/4$	cup water
2	cups powdered sugar
	Decorative colored sugar, optional

Add almond extract, salt, and water to the powdered sugar. Mix until smooth and not too thick. Add a few drops more water if necessary; it needs to be spreading consistency. Spread each cookie with the icing. Sprinkle decorative sugar over each cookie, if desired. Lay cookies out on waxed paper to dry.

Wreath-Shaped Cookies

Use a donut cutter to cut rolled out cookie dough, removing the centers of the circles. Place wreaths on a cookie sheet and bake as directed above. Add a few drops green food coloring to $1/2$ cup grated coconut. Spread the cooled cookie wreaths with icing. Sprinkle coconut on entire surface. Place three red hot candies on each wreath for berries. It is a very pretty cookie.

Store decorated cookies in full size steam table pans or large aluminum foil pans (available at grocery stores), placing one piece of waxed paper in between each layer. Cover the final layer with a lid or foil. Store in a dry place.

The residents enjoyed mixing the dough, cutting out the cookies, and smelling the cookies baking. They also like to decorate the cookies. A pastry brush is a big help to the resident because they do not have to dip the cookie in the frosting and try to flip the cookie over back into its upright position. It is easier to use the pastry brush.

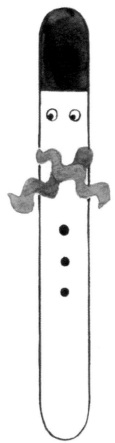

Making a Snowman Ornament

Supplies needed:
>Jumbo craft sticks.
>Clothespins.
>White craft cement.
>White and black acrylic craft paint.
>5mm eyes (peeper).
>Scrap fabric (Christmas material).

Glue 1 clothespin to back of 1 craft stick. Let dry. Paint the whole stick white. Let dry. Paint the top black for a hat. Paint three buttons on tummy. Let dry. Cut thin strip of fabric for a scarf and glue scarf down and eyes on. Let dry. The snowman is completed.

Making a Resident's Christmas Stocking

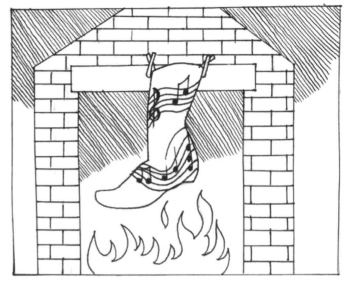

Each stocking is 10$^1/_2$-inches long and is 6-inches across at the foot. The top is 4-inches across.

Supplies needed for each stocking:
1 yard red or green felt.
$^1/_4$ yard white felt.
White craft glue.
Glitter.

For each stocking cut out two pieces of felt in a stocking shape of your choice. Glue edges together with craft glue, leaving the top open. Cut two white pieces of felt to form the top cuff of the stocking and glue onto the top of the stocking on each side. Write the resident's name in with glue and sprinkle the glitter over the glue. I found that if I used a large salt shaker with big holes for the glitter, most residents could shake the glitter over their name. Put on any other designs with the glue and sprinkle the glitter over the glue.

Making Ribbon Christmas Decorations

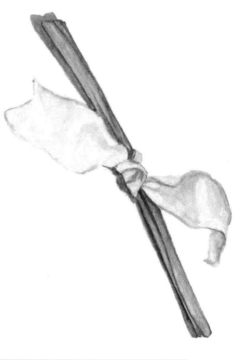

Supplies needed:
1 bolt of 2-inch wide ribbon with wire.
I used ribbon that had green, red, and gold.
Cinnamon sticks in 5-inch and 12-inch lengths.

Cut ribbon in various lengths (12-, 14-, 18-, 24-, and 28-inches). Tie a loose knot in the center of a length of ribbon and tie in a simple bow. Insert one cinnamon stick through the knot of the bow, using the 5-inch cinnamon sticks for the shorter bows and 12-inch sticks for the longer bows. You can use all 12-inch if you desire. It depends on the look you want. These bows are great for table decorations or on Christmas packages.

Using empty boxes, wrap Christmas gifts and use the simple bows on the packages. Place the finished packages under the Christmas tree at facility.

Reflecting on the Meaning of Christmas

Ask the residents the real meaning of Christmas. Encourage the residents to give their opinions of Christmas.

Christmas is reflection.

Christmas is the Christ child.

Christmas is joy.

Christmas is love.

Christmas is a memory.

Christmas is thanksgiving.

Christmas is sharing.

Christmas is a present.

Christmas is a gift.

Christmas is peace on earth and goodwill to man.

Christmas is people, family, and friends.

Christmas is eating your favorite foods.

Christmas is spirit.

Christmas is heart.

Christmas is truth and life.

Christmas is our sovereign King.

Christmas is a blessing.

Christmas is giving thanks to God.

Christmas is being prayerful.

Christmas is the season to be happy.

Christmas is a day to look beyond.

Christmas is singing songs.

Christmas is feasting.

Christmas is a blessing.

Christmas is Christ beside me.

Christmas is music to my ears.

Christmas is faith, hope, and charity.

Christmas is peace.

I went through the above sayings one by one. A few answered and added their own ideas.

Next I played songs and went through some of the words in each song.

"Sing a New Song"

"Joy to the World"

"Come, Sing Out Our Joy"

"Send Out Your Spirit"

"We Walk by Faith"

"The King of Glory"

"Amazing Grace"

"God Sends His Blessing Forth"

"All Good Gifts"

"Let There Be Peace on Earth"

"Taste and See"

"You Are Near"

"Remember Your Love"

"What Shall I Give"

"God Has Chosen Me"

"Deck the Halls"

"Soon and Very Soon"

"Prayer of St. Francis"

"We Have Been Told"

"Where There Is Love"

"Here I Am Lord"

"The King of Love My Shepherd Is"

"The King of Kings, Christ Jesus Reigns"

"God Is Love"

"America the Beautiful"

"How Great Thou Art"

"Lord of All Hopefulness"

"Thanks Be to God"

"In Perfect Charity"

"Come Holy Ghost"

"Crown Him With Many Crowns"

"All People That on Earth Do Dwell"

Reminiscing: Wishing on a Star

Supplies needed: Any items dealing with wishes and stars. I brought:

"Wishing well" wedding box and a bridal card with gift of money.

Birthday cupcake, candle, and birthday picture.

Accordion to play happy birthday to the birthday person.

Picture of child missing two front teeth.

Pennies, water fountain.

Wishbone.

Christmas tree.

A greeting card to wish someone well.

Star items:

> Baseball cap, star glasses, star-patterned note paper, star centerpiece, crown and star wand for a fairy godmother.

Discussion Questions:

Has anyone ever made a wish? What did you wish for? Did your wish come true? Did any of you ever have a wishing well in your garden or yard? What did it look like? Did you ever go to a wedding where a wishing well box was out on the gift table? What was the wishing well box used for at the wedding? Today we have a special resident with a birthday. She is 100 years young. When someone has a birthday what do we say to them? What are some other things we may wish for?

Did you ever wish upon a star? Sing the song "When You Wish Upon a Star." Show the star glasses, baseball cap, and centerpiece. Did you ever wish to go to the moon?

Did your children show off their missing tooth when they were young? Did they put the tooth under their pillow and make a wish for the tooth fairy to come? What did your children receive if they put their tooth under the pillow? Sing "All I Want for Christmas Is My Two Front Teeth."

Does anyone remember the movie "Three Coins in the Fountain"? People often throw pennies in a fountain and make a wish. Let's sing and hum the song "Three Coins in the Fountain." Who would like to throw the pennies into my water fountain and make a wish?

Hold up the wishbone and ask, "What is this called?" Let a resident hold one side of the wishbone and make a wish. Then break the bone apart. Where do wishbones come from? Did you ever save the wishbone from the Thanksgiving turkey? Did you ever make a wish that came true? Can you share your wish?

At Christmas time did you ever wish for a special gift? Do you remember the song, "We Wish You a Merry Christmas"? Let's sing it.

People often buy greeting cards to wish someone happiness or success upon a new baby, job, wedding, or Merry Christmas.

Christmas Wreath Cake

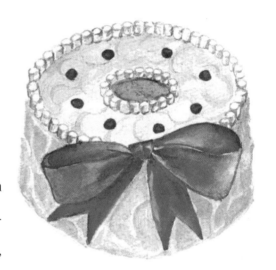

Yield: 12 servings
     1 white cake mix.
     Eggs.
     Oil.
     Water.
     Red and green food coloring.

Preheat oven to 350 degrees. Grease and flour an angel food cake pan. Make a batter with the mix, following the cake mix directions for amounts of eggs, oil, and water. Reserve 1 cup of batter. Pour the remainder of batter into the pan. Divide reserved batter into two bowls. Add a few drops green food coloring to one batch and a few drops red food coloring to the second batch, mixing well. Pour the green and red batter on the top of the white batter in the pan. Swirl in the colored batter with a knife, using a back and forth motion. The cake will be marbled with red and green. Bake for 35-40 minutes or until toothpick inserted in center of cake comes out clean. Cool for about 10 minutes in the pan. Turn the cake out on a plate. Refrigerate cake until cooled completely. Frost with buttercream frosting (recipe on page 295).

Note: *The residents cracked the eggs and mixed the cake mix by hand. It is good exercise for their hands and arms and very good for their self-esteem. They also enjoyed the pretty colors inside the cake. I use an old-fashioned bowl and wooden spoon for the mixing process.*

Buttercream Frosting

$1/2$	cup white margarine
$1/2$	cup shortening
1	pound powdered sugar
1	teaspoon almond extract
$1/4$	teaspoon salt
$1/4$ - $1/3$	cup water
	Green and red food coloring
115-120	miniature marshmallows
9-11	red hots
1	number 104 pastry tip
1	pastry bag

Cream margarine and shortening together. Add powdered sugar, almond extract, and salt. Add $1/4$ cup water and beat until smooth and creamy, adding more water if necessary. Reserve $1/2$ cup of frosting and color it red. Color the remaining frosting green. Frost the entire cake with green frosting. Do not smooth out the frosting but instead swirl the frosting around the cake.

Insert the 104 pastry tip into the pastry bag. Fill bag with red frosting and make a frosting bow at the bottom middle area of the cake.

Place the red hot candies 1- to 2-inches apart in a circle on the top of the cake. Place the miniature marshmallows flat side down around the top outside and inside edges of the cake to act as a border. Some of the residents will not be able to place the red hots or marshmallows but they can watch and visit while taking in the good smells. Some can taste the end product.

I remember making brownies with a couple of the residents on a different occasion. One lady cracked the eggs and mixed up the batter. When her daughter came to visit, her mother told her, "I made brownies." The daughter questioned me. I replied, "Yes, indeed she did. You will have to sample some." It made her daughter feel good, too. It also gave the resident a sense of pride.

A Winter Nature Walk

Supplies needed:

Branches from several varieties of evergreen. I brought:

Colorado blue spruce.

Scotch pine.

White pine.

Norway spruce.

Mugho pine.

Balsam fir.

Columnar arborvita.

Hetzi juniper.

Pyramidal arborvita.

Andora juniper.

Seagreen juniper.

Pinecones.

Pinecone wreath.

Wreath made of straw.

I sat the group around a round table to view the branches one at a time. I told them the names and passed the branches around the table for the residents to see, touch, and smell. It doesn't matter that they can't name the trees. They can touch and smell the branches. Some of them remembered the Norway spruce because they had them growing in their yards.

New Year's Eve Day Party

We decorated the room New Year's style with streamers, bells, whistles, noisemakers, and hats. Each resident got a hat and a noisemaker.

The party and entertainment began at 11:00 a.m. We danced with the residents in their wheelchairs. We sang patriotic songs. In addition I played polka music and strolled around the room with my accordion. Just before noon we had a countdown: 10, 9, 8… and at the stroke of noon, yelled "Happy New Year!" Shortly after noon the kitchen served a lunch party consisting of shrimp, meatballs, chicken wings, vegetables, cheese, crackers, salad, and bread.

This party was simple for the activity department to put together yet relaxing for the residents. Lunch was an excellent time for we were able to get most of the residents to participate in this activity.

So now you can enjoy reading this book and implementing these ideas into your programs at your facility.
Remember to work with your residents in their world, at their pace. Live for the moment. Relax and laugh with them. Have fun!

Best Wishes,
Pat Nekola

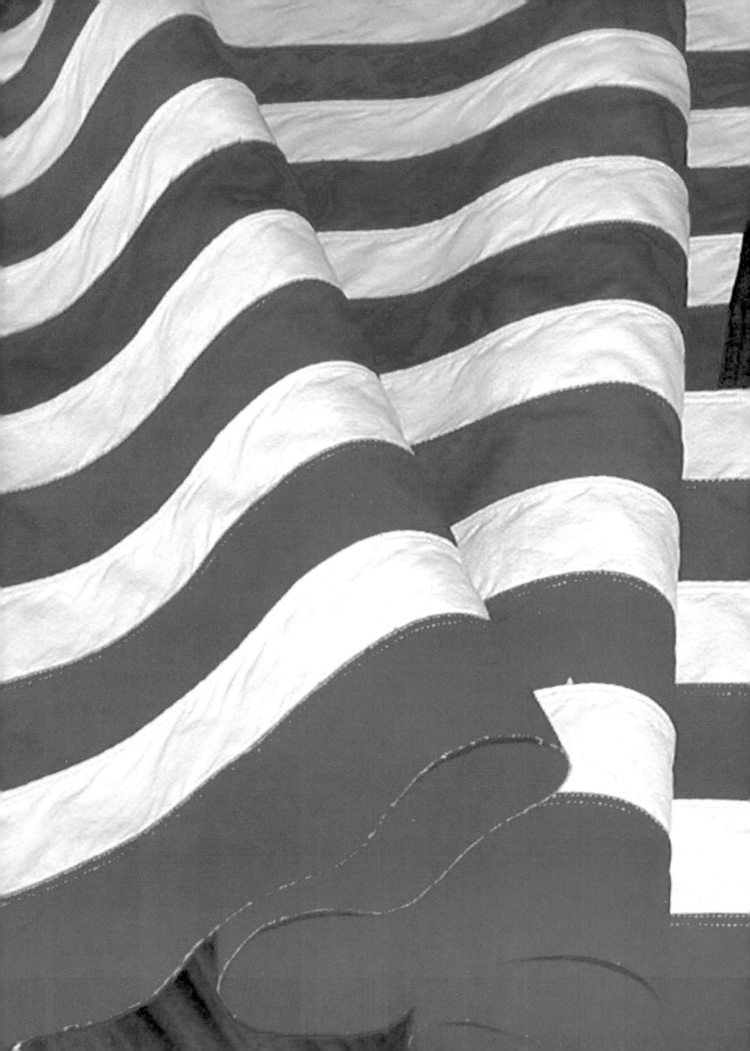

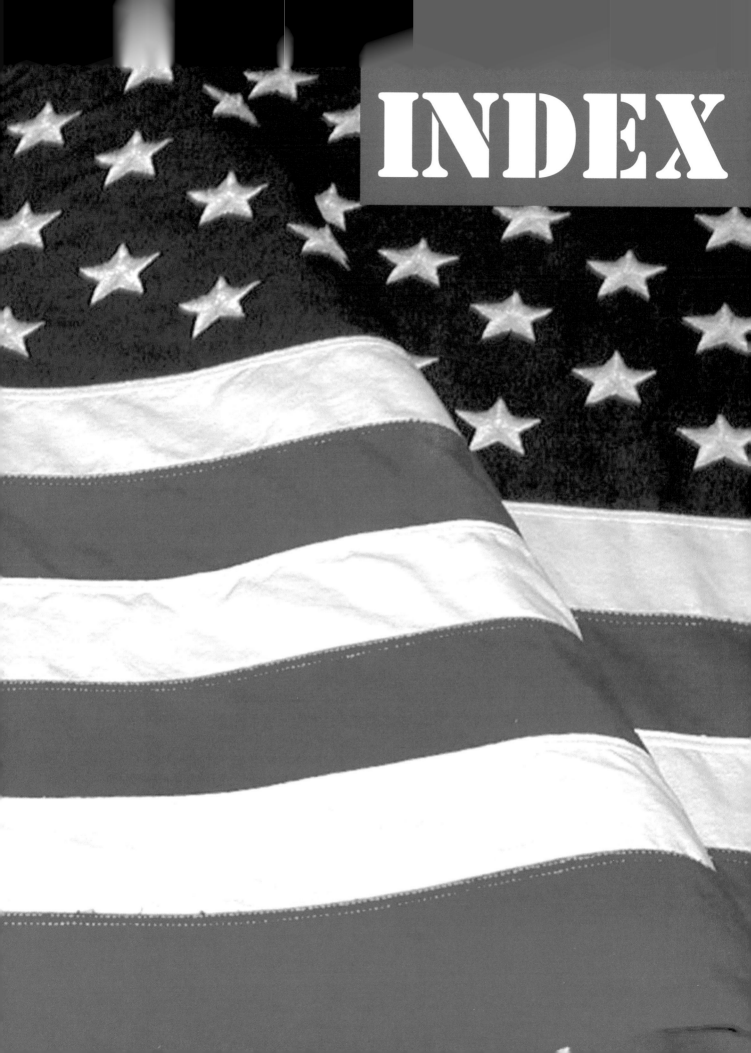

INDEX

■

Index

Website Directory

Alzheimer's Association: . . . . www.alz.org/

Assisted Living Federation of America: . . . .(email) info@alfa.org or (website) www.alfa.org

Author Pat Nekola:. . . . . www.patnekolabooks.com

Medicare: . . . . www.medicare.gov

National Certification Council of Activity Professionals: . . . . www.nccap.org

National Kidney Foundation: . . . . www.kidney.org

Social Security Administration (SSA): . . . . www.ssa.gov

Children of Aging Parents: www.caps4caregivers.org

Telephone Number Directory

Alzheimer's Association, Chicago
. . . .(312) 335-8700 or (800) 272-3900

Alzheimer's Disease Education and Referral
Center (ADEAR) . . . . (800) 438-4380

American Association of Retired Persons
(AARP) . . . (202) 434-2277 or (800) 424-3410

Area Agency On Aging
(AAA) . . . . (202) 296-8130

Assisted Living Federation of America
. . . . (703) 691-8100 or 1-800-227-7294

Elder Abuse Hotline (national numbers) (800) 677-1116

Eldercare Locator . . . . (800) 677-1116

Insurance Consumer Helpline . . . . (800) 942-4242

Medicaid, Wisconsin . . . . (800) 362-3002

Medicare . . . . (800) 633-4227
Hard of Hearing . . . . (877) 486-2048

National Association for Continence
. . . . (800) 252-3337

National Certification Council of Activity
Professionals . . . . (757) 552-0653

National Council on the Aging Inc.
. . . .(202) 479-1200

National Hospice Organization . . . . (800) 658-8898

National Institute on Aging . . . . . . (301) 496-1752

National Kidney Foundation . . . . . (800) 622-9010

Railroad Retirement Board . . . . . . (800) 808-0772

Social Security Administration . . . (800) 772-1213
Hard of Hearing . . . . (800) 325-0778

Social Security Administration Fraud Hotline
. . . .(800) 269-0271

Veteran's Administration . . . . (800) 827-1000

Wisconsin Geriatric Education Center
. . . .(414) 288-3712

Picnics

Catering on the Move:
A Cookbook and Guide
by Pat Nekola

Learn to cater your own picnic for family and friends, for church or service club gatherings, or open a catering business. This cookbook has a variety of recipes designed especially for picnics. View buffet layouts, decorations, and various styles of picnics from simple to elegant. Recipes serve groups of 12-100, some up to 1,500!

Snacks and beverages, salads, grilled meats, hot vegetables, and desserts recipes are all designed for the picnicker's appetite.

From the owner of Pat's Party Foods, Caterers.

242 pages, hard back with spiral binding.
ISBN: 0-9660610-0-4
February 2000, Catering by Design

Pat Nekola has a long history of fine catering with her own business, Pat's Party Foods, in Wisconsin. She cooked many delicious recipes in *Picnics, Catering on the Move*. Picnics were her favorite parties because she enjoyed watching families and friends relax and have fun.

Pat Nekola began writing *Picnics, Catering on the Move* when her mother was diagnosed with Alzheimer's disease. Alzheimer's is a progressive, degenerative disease of the brain causing confusion, personality, and behavioral changes. Eventually many people with Alzheimer's are not able to care for themselves. A family member loses them twice: first to Alzheimer's, then to death. Taking care of a person with Alzheimer's takes a lot of patience and love.

Pat is donating $3.00 of every book sold to the Alzheimer's Association. The funds are being used for research to find a cure for the disease and for educational programs that help caregivers.

- *Kitchen-tested recipes.*
- *Picnic ideas.*
- *Quantities shown for small to large groups.*
- *Decorations for theme parties.*
- *Diagrams to guide the reader.*
- *Buffet layout diagrams act as a learning tool.*
- *Heartwarming stories accompany recipes.*
- *Easy-to-follow instructions.*
- *Garnishes to make food attractive.*
- *Catering for crowds for fun and profit.*

Picnics
Catering on the Move:
A Cookbook and Guide
by Pat Nekola

Customer Name _____
Library _____
Address _____
City State Zip _____
Phone _____ Fax _____

Mail or fax to:	**Catering by Design** P.O. Box 181 Waukesha, WI 53187 Ph: (262) 547-2004 Fax: (262) 547-8594

Qty:	Price @	Ext.
	$27.95	$
Shipping	$4.35	$
Total		$

Terms: 30 days

Signature _____

Date _____

Invoice Number _____

Thank you for your order!